CLARE MAXWELL-HUDSON'S

AROMATHERAPY
MASSAGE

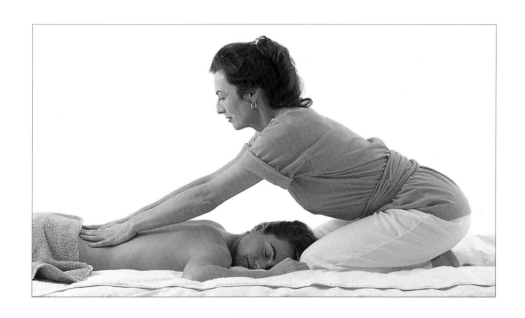

A DK PUBLISHING BOOK

Massage Photography Sandra Lousada

Art Editor Jo Grey
Project Editor Helen Townsend
Designer Helen Diplock
D.T.P. Designer Karen Ruane

Senior Art Editor Tracy Timson
Senior Editor Susannah Marriott

Managing Art Editor Carole Ash
Managing Editor Rosie Pearson
Production Manager Maryann Rogers

U.S. Editor Mary Ann Lynch

This book is dedicated to my mother

Important Notice

Refer to the safety precautions on page 16 before using any essential oil.
Do not try self-treatment during pregnancy, or for serious or long-term
problems, without consulting a doctor. Seek medical advice if symptoms
persist. Neither the author nor the publisher can be held responsible for any
damage, injury, or otherwise resulting from the use of any essential oils.

First American edition, 1994
First paperback edition, 1997
2 4 6 8 10 9 7 5 3 1

Published in the United States by DK Publishing, Inc.,
95 Madison Avenue, New York, NY 10016
Visit us on the World Wide Web at http://www.dk.com

Library of Congress Cataloging-in-Publication Data

Maxwell-Hudson, Clare.
    Aromatherapy massage : the complete illustrated guide to
massaging with essential oils / Clare Maxwell-Hudson.
       p.   cm.
    Includes index.
    ISBN 1-56458-642-1 (hardcover)
    ISBN 0-7894-1654-9 (paper back)
    1. Aromatherapy.   I. Title
RM666.A68M39 1994   94-16051
615'.321--dc20   CIP

Reproduced by Colourscan, Singapore
Printed in Great Britain by Butler and Tanner

CONTENTS

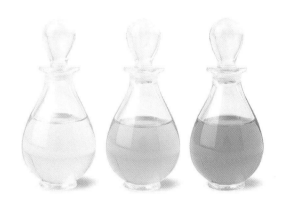

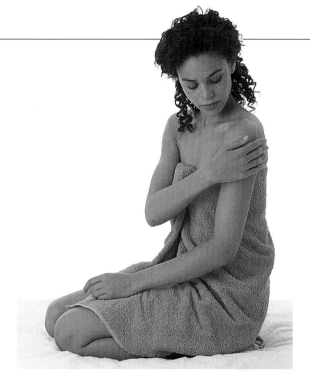

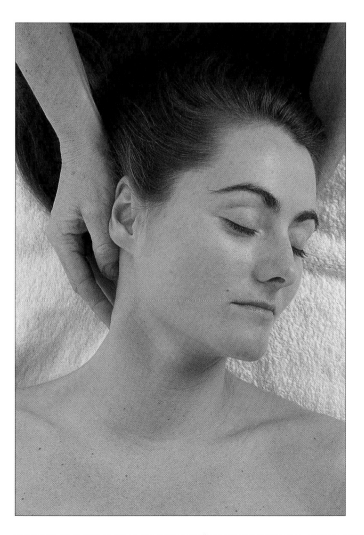

INTRODUCTION

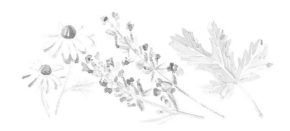

FRAGRANT ESSENTIAL OILS can enrich your life, whether they are used therapeutically, in beauty treatments, to perfume the home, or for sheer pleasure. But when the oils are combined with massage, their effectiveness in relieving stress, improving mood, and promoting good health is most striking.

WHAT IS AROMATHERAPY?

"Aroma" derives from the Greek word for spice – today we use the word more broadly to mean fragrance – and "therapy" means treatment, so aromatherapy literally means curative treatment by the use of scent. My research into the therapeutic properties of essential oils and the plants from which they derive has led me all over the world and brought me into contact with many cultures in which essential oils are valued. In *Aromatherapy Massage,* I reveal the traditional healing qualities attributed to my favorite oils and discuss the properties ascribed to them by the latest research. I have always used essential oils to create oil blends in the belief that they enhance the effects of a massage. Odors are perceived by the part of the brain connected with emotion, and research has shown that a pleasurable scent can have a positive effect on your enjoyment of life.

THE ART OF MASSAGE

Massage is probably the oldest and simplest of medical treatments. Rubbing an aching shoulder or soothing a furrowed brow is a healing instinct common to all cultures. Over two thousand years ago, the Greek physician Hippocrates said, "Rubbing can bind a joint that is too loose and loosen a joint that is too rigid." This is the most fascinating part of massage: the same strokes can produce so many different effects. Brisk movements invigorate, while similar movements performed slowly can induce sleep. And, because massage is almost second nature, the techniques are easy to learn. The physical benefits of massage, such as improved circulation and relaxed muscles, and the psychological feelings of being comforted and cared for, produce a sense of well-being that is surely unique.

TOUCH & SCENT

Aromatherapy massage is an art that involves an intimate interaction between the person giving the massage and the person receiving it, and the aroma of the oils. Each blend of oils is personalized, determined both by the scents the recipient prefers and by their desired effect – whether it is to relieve minor ailments, to pamper with an aromatic beauty treatment, or simply to ease tension with a full body massage.

Over 700 years ago, Rumi, an Afghan poet and philosopher, related the benefits of aromatherapy in this story: Once upon a time, there was a man who had an illness that none seemed able to cure. After much traveling, he found a very wise doctor who gave him a stick and told him to go for a walk with it every day. A month later, the man was completely cured. He returned to the doctor, who revealed that the handle of the stick was filled with aromatic plants and spices, and the heat and rubbing of the man's hand released their healing properties. I hope that aromatherapy will have the same beneficial effect for you, and that *Aromatherapy Massage* will help you experience touch and smell in the most pleasurable way – through giving and receiving massage with scented oils.

Clare Maxwell-Hudson

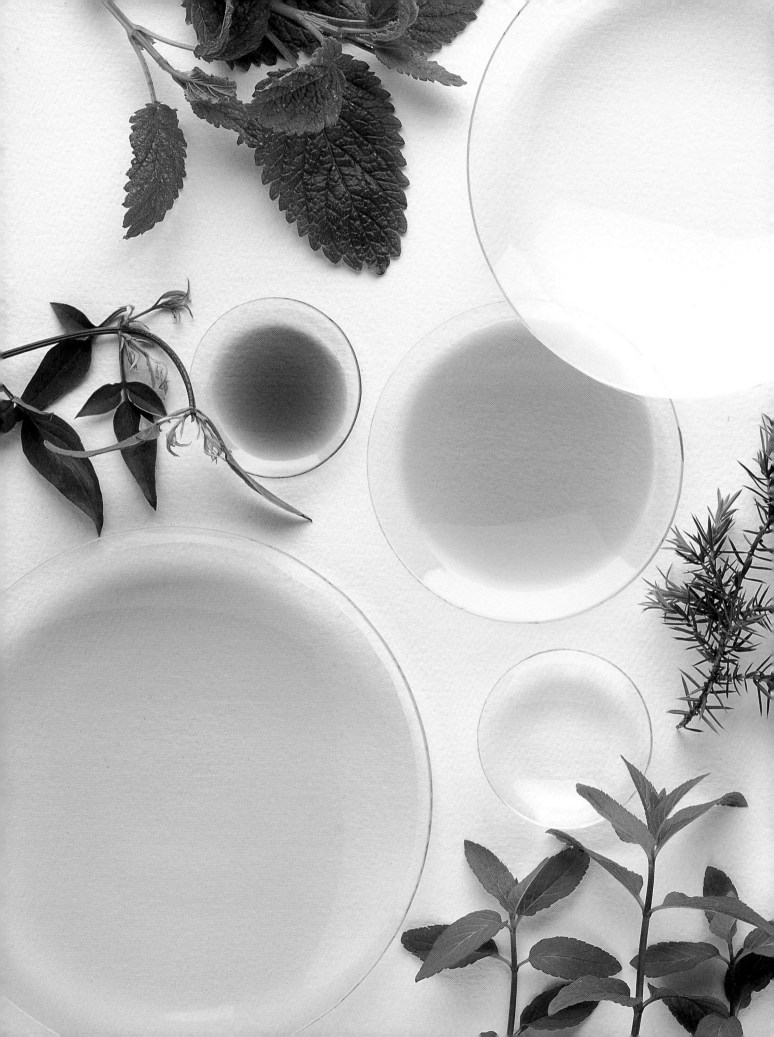

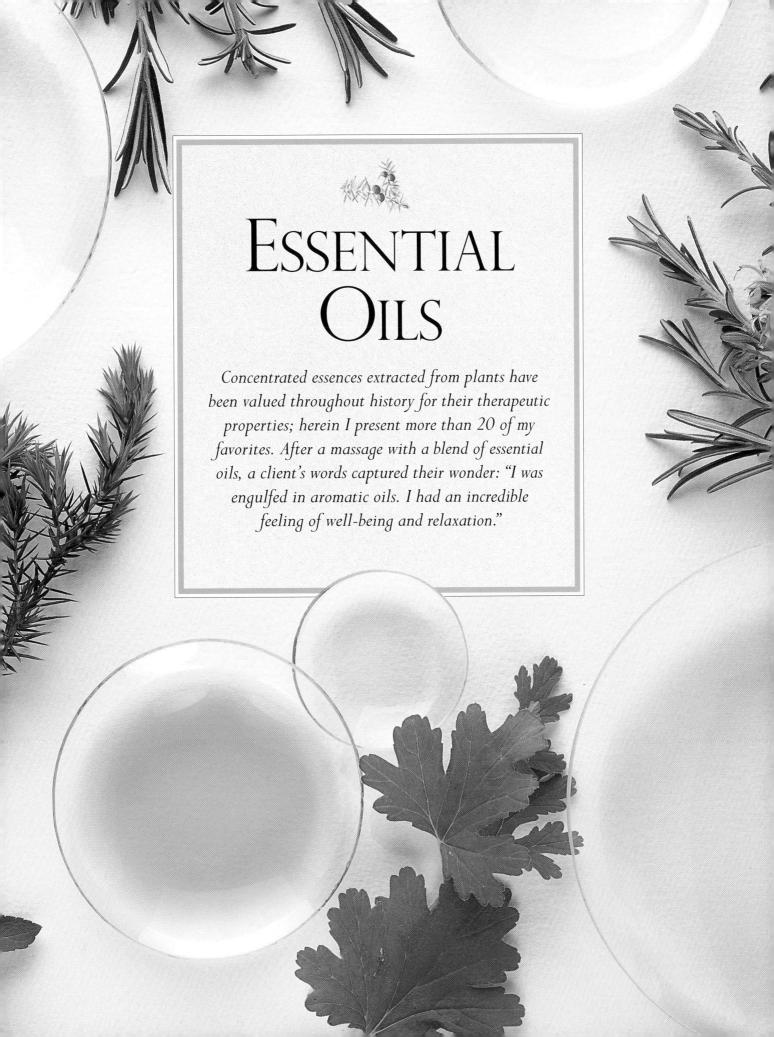

ESSENTIAL OILS

Concentrated essences extracted from plants have been valued throughout history for their therapeutic properties; herein I present more than 20 of my favorites. After a massage with a blend of essential oils, a client's words captured their wonder: "I was engulfed in aromatic oils. I had an incredible feeling of well-being and relaxation."

AROMATHERAPY IN HISTORY

Numerous powers have been attributed to fragrant plants, and they have been used throughout history in the pursuit of happiness and health: as part of medicine, religion, and magic; and in cosmetics. In early civilizations, scented woods and oils were often burned to communicate with gods or to exorcise demons, and even today incense is part of many religious ceremonies. Massage with aromatic oils also softens and perfumes the skin and aids healing.

MASTER PERFUMERS

The Ancient Egyptians greatly appreciated fragrance, and wealthy men and women used scented oils daily in massage to soften and protect their skin from the harsh, dry climate. Cleopatra is even said to have seduced Mark Antony with fragrance, by covering the floors 18 inches deep in rose petals.

The Egyptians also had a sophisticated knowledge of the antiseptic properties of aromatic plants and oils, using them to embalm the dead. Ointments found in Tutankhamun's tomb, dating from *c.*1320BC, were found to contain frankincense, gum resins, and spikenard and, remarkably, still retained their scent.

The Ancient Greeks learned about fragrance from the Egyptians, whom they revered as master perfumers. Believing aromatics enabled them to drink more wine, wealthy Athenians placed bags of fragrant flowers and vases of unguents on their banquet tables. Scented oils were also used for massage and were thought to have medicinal properties – the lyric poet Anacreon (582–*c.*485BC) claimed "The best recipe for health is to apply sweet scents to the brain."

The Romans developed public baths, believing in their health-giving properties, and bathing was followed by scented massage. Barbers soothed men's faces with hot towels and scented oils, and wealthy women refreshed their bodies with rosewater. The knowledge of the healing properties of plants spread with the Romans, and in the 2nd century, Galen, physician to Marcus Aurelius, wrote on many branches of medicine and taught the benefits of massage. He also invented cold cream by adding water to an ointment, which cooled the skin as the water evaporated (see page 79).

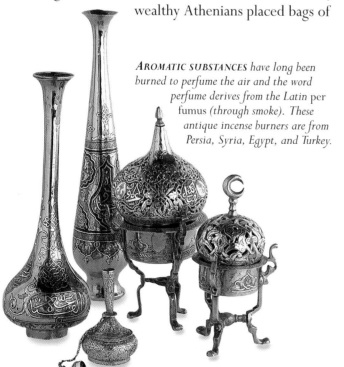

AROMATIC SUBSTANCES have long been burned to perfume the air and the word perfume derives from the Latin per fumus (through smoke). These antique incense burners are from Persia, Syria, Egypt, and Turkey.

FRAGRANCES OF ASIA

Aromatic oils have been used in Chinese herbalism for thousands of years – an important herbal from around 200BC, which is named after the legendary Shen Nong, lists 365 plants used medicinally.

Throughout Asia, perfumes have always been prized for their medicinal and cosmetic properties: a still found in the Himalayan foothills indicates that the distillation of essential oils prospered in 3000BC, and in modern bazaars from Istanbul to Bombay, oils and aromatic remedies are abundant. In the 9th century Baghdad, in what is now Iraq, was the center of the rose industry and thrived on the export of rosewater to India. Avicenna, a philosopher and physician born in 980 in Bukhara, in what is now Uzbekistan, is credited with improving the rose distillation process through his invention of the refrigerated coil. He also

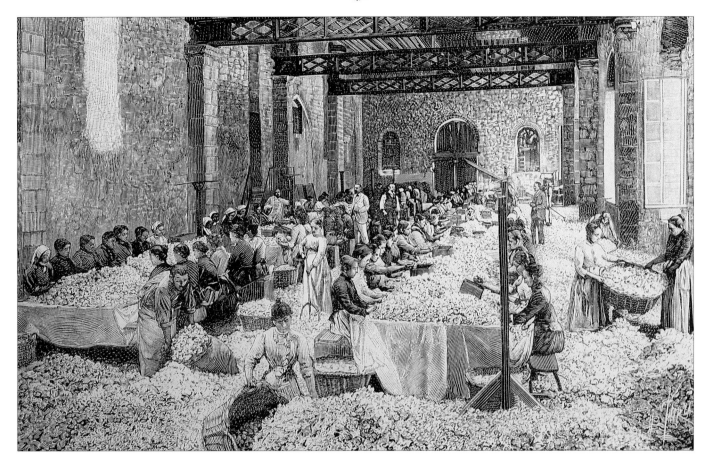

wrote numerous books on health, including the *Kitab al-Qanun*, or *Canon of Medicine*, in which the action of medicinal and aromatic plants and spices was explored.

India has a long tradition of using aromatic plants, and the holistic system of Ayurvedic medicine, which views health as a balance between person and environment, often combines scented oils and spices with massage.

ESSENTIAL OILS IN EUROPE

With the influence of the Crusades in the 12th century, trade routes had developed with the Middle East, bringing an influx of spices, herbs, and exotic scents. Herb gardens were cultivated in monasteries, and monks and nuns prepared popular remedies such as Carmelite water made with melissa. From the Middle Ages on, numerous herbals, categorizing plants and their therapeutic remedies, were compiled, including those of herbalists Nicholas Culpeper (1652), William Turner (1568), and John Gerard (1597).

In the 18th century, aromatic vinegars and perfumed waters gained greatly in popularity, especially eau de cologne. This product was a favorite of the Emperor Napoleon and considered to be an elixir of life. Four

THIS ENGRAVING from 1898 shows the commercial production of rose oil, which began in Grasse in the south of France in the 18th century.

grave-robbers from Marseilles had earlier won notoriety for a vinegar recipe that they claimed protected them from the plague (see page 84).

In the early 20th century, Réné Gattefossé, a French chemist working in his family perfumery, became fascinated by the therapeutic properties of essential oils when, after burning his hands, he rinsed them with lavender essence, which stopped "the gasification of the tissues." He studied the antiseptic, bactericidal, antiviral, and anti-inflammatory properties of essential oils, and in 1937 introduced the term *aromatherapie*.

During World Wars I and II, essential oils were used to treat wounds, and in the 1960s, Dr. Jean Valnet, one of the French doctors who pioneered this work, published his findings on essential oils. Austrian biochemist Marguerite Maury studied Valnet's work and introduced aromatherapy to Britain. She continued research into the benefits of essential oils for health and beauty, created the concept of the individual prescription (see page 15), and rekindled the ancient link between aromatherapy and massage.

HARVESTING & EXTRACTION

Essential oils, occasionally referred to as essences, volatile oils, or ethereal oils, are highly concentrated substances extracted from aromatic plants that are commercially cultivated throughout the world. Turkey and Bulgaria are famous for rose oil, India for jasmine, and the island of Réunion for geranium, while tea tree oil is associated with Australia and mint with the U.S. However, the essential oil industry is subject to the vagaries of climate and to political upheaval, and the sources of specific oils have changed many times throughout history.

CLIMATE & HARVESTING

The production of essential oils can be variable, but on average, 154 lb (70 kg) of plant material produces around 4¼ pints (2 liters) of essential oil. Because plants are at the mercy of weather and soil conditions, their yield and quality varies from year to year. In 1970, for instance, the geranium crop of Réunion was destroyed by a cyclone. Réunion's inability to supply the oil led to a shortage, causing the price to increase, which in turn prompted other countries, among them Egypt, to cultivate geraniums. The yield of essential oil also depends on the time of harvesting. Certain plants, such as ylang ylang, are picked early in the morning when they are most aromatic. Others, including jasmine, are harvested at night, when their scent is strongest. Some plants, such as the rose, are processed at the source so as not to lose any volatile oils, while others, such as juniper, must first be dried and can then be exported for distillation.

EXTRACTION

Steam distillation is the most common method of extraction. Plant material is heated by steam in a still, and the volatile parts present in the plant evaporate into the steam. These vapors are carried along a closed outlet and are cooled and condensed by being passed through a cold-water jacket. The resulting water is collected in a flask, where the essential oil floats on the surface. Flower water is a by-product.
In solvent extraction, plant material is placed in a drum with a hydrocarbon solvent to dissolve the essential oil. The solution is filtered off and concentrated by distillation, leaving behind either a "concrete," a combination of wax and essential oil, or

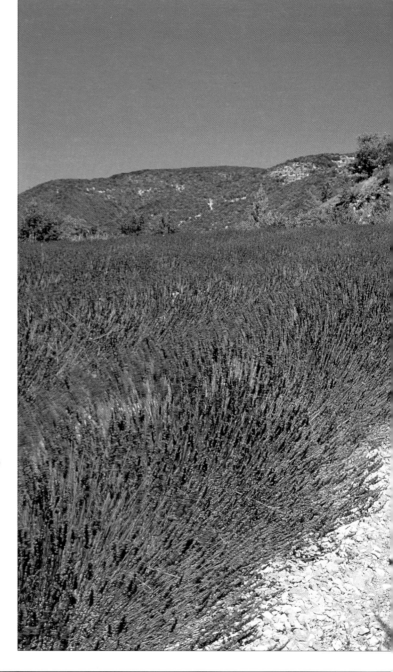

a "resinoid," a substance containing resin. A second process of solvent extraction using pure alcohol recovers most of the oil. The alcohol is then evaporated, leaving a solution called "absolute."

The phytonic process is a new, highly efficient and economical form of solvent extraction developed in Britain by Dr. Peter Wilde. Environmentally friendly solvents are used at room temperature in a sealed apparatus to extract essential oil, "phytol," from plants.

Super-critical carbon dioxide extraction uses carbon dioxide gas at very high pressure to dissolve essential oil from a wide range of plant materials. The equipment is massive and extremely expensive, but there are several process plants around the world producing essential oils of excellent quality.

Expression is a process used to extract essential oil from citrus fruits. The rind of the fruit is crushed to release the essential oil just under the surface.

Enfleurage, now nearly obsolete, involved pressing flowers into fat-coated glass plates. The flowers were replaced daily until the fat was saturated with essential oil, which was then dissolved from the fat with alcohol.

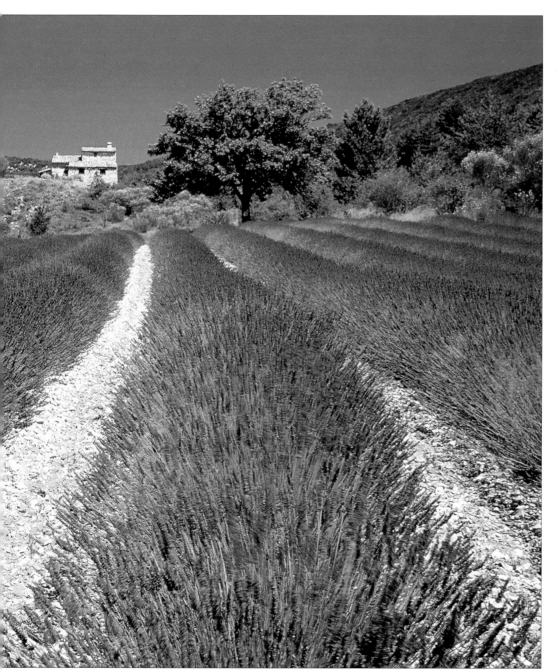

TODAY, LAVENDER FIELDS are usually harvested by slow-moving machines. They begin picking the flowers early in the morning and continue throughout the day. Roughly 440 lb (200 kg) of lavender flowers are needed to produce about 12¾ pints (6 liters) of essential oil, using the process of steam distillation.

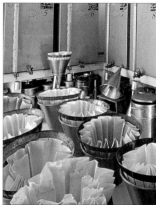

A TRADITIONAL PROCESS of extraction, known as maceration and filtration, is employed at the Fragonard perfumery in Grasse, France. Plant material is placed in hot oil, which absorbs the plant's aromatic essence. The plant material is removed and the process is repeated until the oil is perfumed.

CARRIER OILS & BLENDING

Carrier oils are used to dilute essential oils for use in aromatherapy massage and to make beauty preparations. Containing vitamins, proteins, and minerals, they are highly effective moisturizers and provide many of the nutrients that the skin needs to keep it smooth and supple. Cold-pressed carrier oils are usually of a higher quality than heat- or solvent-extracted oils.

ALL-PURPOSE CARRIER OILS

These viscous oils can be used alone, or, when enriched with special oils, used to dilute essential oils for use in aromatherapy massage, cosmetics, or a fragrant bath.

Apricot kernel oil, extracted from the apricot kernel, is rich in minerals and vitamins. A natural moisturizer, it has a light texture and high penetrative qualities.
Sunflower oil is a lovely fine oil that I use in most of my blends for body massage. It contains vitamin E.
Soy oil, extracted from the soy bean plant, is light, nourishing, easily absorbed, and especially suited to oily skin.
Sweet almond oil is extracted from the almond kernel and has soothing, softening properties. Always use the sweet, not bitter, variety. Popular throughout history, sweet almond oil is also suitable for babies.
Grapeseed oil, extracted from the seeds of muscat raisins by heat, is good for oily skin.

SPECIAL CARRIER OILS

These special oils can be added to all-purpose oils to create a long-lasting, more absorbent blend that is good for nourishing dry, dehydrated skin.

Carrot oil is rich in vitamins, especially A. Add only 10% to other carrier oils, because its bright orange color can temporarily stain the skin.
Sesame oil, extracted from the raw sesame seed, has a slightly nutty aroma and contains 85% unsaturated and 15% saturated fatty acids. It can be added to other oils to enrich them. Do not use the heavy-scented brown oil from the cooked seed.
Avocado oil is extracted from the flesh of the avocado. It is rich in vitamins A and B, and in lecithin, proteins, and fatty acids. An excellent skin softener, it is easily absorbed.

Jojoba is a natural liquid wax from the kernels of an evergreen desert plant and has a chemical composition resembling the skin's sebum. Jojoba's waxy structure and anti-bacterial properties give it a long shelf life. Readily absorbed by the skin, it has a non-oily softening effect and is especially suitable for the face. It is also good for thickening creams.
Wheat-germ oil is rich and viscous, but its strong smell can be difficult to mask. Add 10-20% wheat-germ oil to other carrier oils to guard against rancidity and prolong the life of a blend.

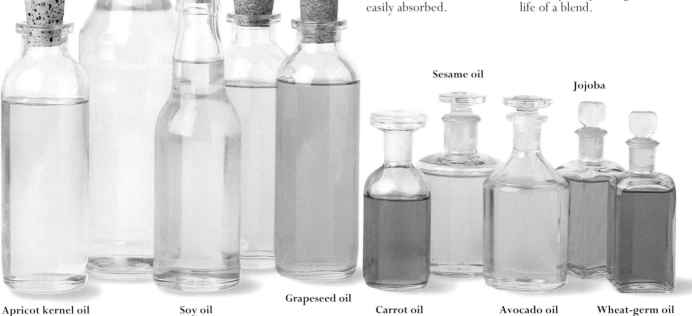

Sunflower oil

Sweet almond oil

Sesame oil

Jojoba

Apricot kernel oil

Soy oil

Grapeseed oil

Carrot oil

Avocado oil

Wheat-germ oil

Choosing Essential Oils

An oil blend is made by mixing a few drops of essential oil with one of the carrier oils opposite. We all like different scents, and it is essential that the aroma of the blend appeals to you, or to the person you are going to massage. Create what Marguerite Maury (see page 11) called "an individual prescription." First, decide what effect you hope to achieve: do you want the aroma to sedate or revive, to energize or to calm? Do you want to use oils for their therapeutic properties or simply to pamper? Then, referring to pages 17–39, make a list of essential oils suited to your requirements. Select two or three from your list – good blends usually combine all three notes: top (gives the initial scent), middle (adds body to the blend), and base (released last, this gives the lingering scent). The general rule is that a little is best: a weak blend of oils often smells better and is therefore more effective than a stronger blend. Follow the guide below to achieve the safest dilution of essential oils for a balanced fragrance and maximum therapeutic benefit.

Blending Oils

Oil blends are usually divided into normal and low dilutions. Aromatherapists refer to these dilutions as percentages, based on the amount of essential oil in carrier oil. There is an easy way to figure out dilutions. To calculate how many drops of essential oil are needed to make a normal dilution of 2½%, divide the number of milliliters of carrier oil by 2; for a low dilution of 1%, divide by 4. Most essential oil bottles come with a dropper for easy measuring. Refer to the individual essential oil entries on pages 17–39, paying special attention to the warnings listed, for special instructions on which dilution to use. For a full body massage, 20ml of oil is needed; for the face, 10 ml is enough. You can make larger quantities and store them (see page 16).

MAKING AN OIL BLEND

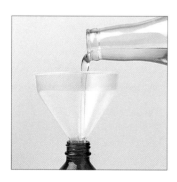

1 Choose a carrier oil (or blend of carrier oils) based on your skin type, and determine the amount you will need. Transfer the carrier oil into a dark bottle a little larger than the amount of oil.

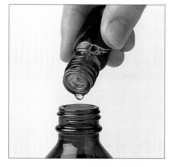

2 Choose 2–3 essential oils based on the effect you require, and calculate the number of drops to use. Add to the carrier oil. Close the bottle and label it clearly. Shake well before use.

BLENDING GUIDE

Normal dilution of 2½%:

ml carrier oil ÷ 2 = total drops essential oil
(e.g. 20 ml carrier oil ÷ 2 = 10 drops essential oil)

SAMPLE 2½% BLEND

Essential Oils
5 drops sandalwood
3 drops lavender
2 drops orange
Carrier Oil
20 ml apricot kernel

TOTAL: 10 drops essential oil per 20 ml carrier oil

**Low dilution of 1% for sensitive skin
and for use during pregnancy:**

ml carrier oil ÷ 4 = total drops essential oil
(e.g. 20 ml carrier oil ÷ 4 = 5 drops essential oil)

SAMPLE 1% BLEND

Essential Oils
3 drops rosemary
1 drop each of lemongrass and juniper
Carrier Oil
20 ml sunflower oil

TOTAL: 5 drops essential oil per 20 ml carrier oil

**Extremely low dilution for very sensitive
skin, children & babies:**

Use just 1 drop essential oil per 10 ml carrier oil, or use sweet almond oil by itself.

STORAGE & SAFETY

It is a common misconception that anything natural is safe. Yet many dangerous poisons are natural, and almost anything used in excess can be harmful. Since essential oils are highly concentrated, they need to be used with care. Before you start to use essential oils, read these guidelines to ensure that your oil blends and treatments will be successful and enjoyable.

STORAGE

Essential oils are highly volatile and evaporate easily. As heat, air, and light affect them, they should be kept in dark glass bottles in normal to cool temperatures (65°F/18°C). Although some wood oils can improve with age, most oils slowly deteriorate and should be used within a couple of years. They can be stored in the bottom of the refrigerator to prolong their life. Do not worry if they solidify – they will liquefy at room temperature. Citrus oils should be used within a year. Once the essential oils have been diluted in a carrier oil, their shelf life is reduced to a few months.

LABEL all oil blends

STORAGE GUIDELINES

• Store oils in dark glass bottles in a cool, dark place with the lids tightly secured to prevent evaporation

• Label bottles with the oils, dilution, and date

• Store out of reach of children

• Essential oils are flammable, so keep them away from open flames

• Do not store on polished surfaces, since the oils can leave marks; wipe up spills immediately.

PATCH TEST
Place a drop of diluted essential oil (2½%) on the inside of your wrist or the crease of your elbow. Cover with a bandage and examine after 12 hours. If there is any redness or itching, do not use the oil. If you have an adverse reaction to an oil, apply sweet almond oil to the area, then wash with cold water.

SAFETY

Essential oils should always be diluted. It is possible to irritate the skin by using too strong a concentration of oil. To avoid possible irritation or allergic reaction, do a patch test (see below, left) before using a new essential oil on yourself or a friend, and adhere strictly to the recommended dilutions (see page 15).

SAFETY PRECAUTIONS

• Keep essential oils away from children and pets

• Never take essential oils internally unless prescribed by a medically qualified aromatherapist

• Do not apply oils to the skin neat. The only exception is spot application of one drop of lavender or tea tree oil using a cotton swab for stings, pimples, or cuts

• Do not rub your eyes after using essential oils; if oil gets in the eye, rinse at once with cool water

• During pregnancy, consult a doctor and qualified aromatherapist since some oils should be avoided; use low dilutions (1% or less) of gentle oils such as chamomile, citrus oils, frankincense, geranium, lavender, sandalwood, and rose

• If you have epilepsy, consult a doctor before using essential oils; check the warnings for each oil before use, because some are stimulants

• Use the recommended mild oils (see pages 19, 20, and 31) for young children in extremely low dilutions (1% or less), and consult a qualified aromatherapist

• For sensitive skin, use well-diluted oils (1%)

• Citrus oils increase sensitivity to the sun, so avoid sun and sunlamps for six hours after use

• If taking homeopathic medicine, consult a homeopath before using essential oils; oils may reduce effectiveness

• Avoid prolonged use of the same essential oil.

A CATALOG OF OILS

An illustrated catalog of more than 20 of my favorite essential oils follows, arranged in alphabetical order by the botanical names of the plants from which the oils are derived. The catalog includes photographs of the plant source and essential oil, plus details of scent, expense, "note," and chemical constituents. Historical anecdotes and the latest scientific research with details of the main therapeutic uses are covered, and a suitable massage and compatible oils for use in blends are suggested. Key information is listed and explained below.

USING THE CATALOG

① BOTANICAL NAME
Sometimes more than one name appears, since certain essential oils have more than one plant source.

② THERAPEUTIC PROPERTIES
This is a guide to traditional uses of essential oils and modern scientific research. It is divided into sections that explain how the oils are used, with cross-references to more practical sections of the book.

③ OIL COMBINATIONS
Three complementary oils are suggested for use in an oil blend to enhance the essential oil featured.

④ SCENT
This describes the fragrance of the essential oil.

⑤ NOTES
In *The Art of Perfumery* (1862), Septimus Piesse classified scents as musical notes. Top notes are the first impressions of a scent, middle notes are the body, and base notes are fragrances that last. One oil can have all three notes; some have one or two and do not last long; the color bar varies from weak to strong to reflect the intensity of the notes.

⑥ EXPENSE RATING
One star indicates the least expensive oil, and four stars the most expensive. The price reflects the yield of oil in the plant, but it does not guarantee quality. Trust your sense of smell and the integrity of your supplier.

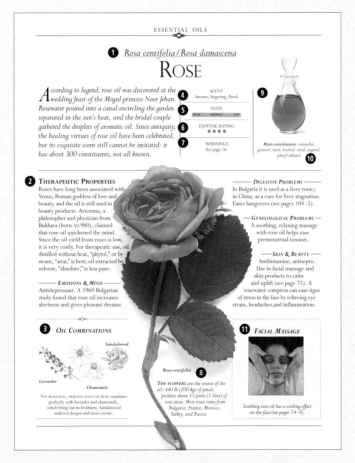

⑦ WARNINGS
Any warnings unique to a particular oil are stated here, but before using any essential oil, read the safety information on page 16.

⑧ PLANT SOURCE
The plant from which the oil is extracted is shown, noting which part is used and how the oil is extracted.

⑨ COLOR RANGE
Essential oils vary from clear to dark blue to bright orange.

⑩ MAIN CONSTITUENTS
Essential oils have a complex chemical make-up, and not all elements have been identified. The main constituents include terpenes and their derivatives (alcohols, esters, aldehydes, ketones, phenols). These feature widely in essential oils. Oils with high levels of alcohols and esters, such as clary sage, have gentle, healing properties. Aldehydes, ketones, and phenols are therapeutically active, but oils with these constituents, such as lemongrass, should be used in low concentrations. Of the other constituents, monoterpenes, including camphene and limonene, have antiviral properties, while sesquiterpenes are less volatile and have a stronger odor.

⑪ SUITABLE MASSAGE
A massage is suggested for a part of the body where the oil is especially effective.

Boswellia carterii / Boswellia thurifera
FRANKINCENSE

The earliest record of frankincense is a relief in a magnificent temple in Upper Egypt, built in the 15th century BC by Queen Hatshepsut. The relief illustrates an expedition to Punt, on the coast of modern-day Somalia, to collect this precious gum. Frankincense was used extensively in temple rituals, and as a perfume and medicine. It is a key element of incense and plays a part in holy rituals today.

SCENT
Balsamic, rich, sweet, warm

NOTE
| BASE | MIDDLE | TOP |

EXPENSE RATING
✳✳

WARNINGS
See page 16.

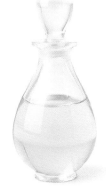

Main constituents:
monoterpenes, olibanol, pinene, camphene, limonene, resinous substances

THERAPEUTIC PROPERTIES

Frankincense, called olibanum in the Arabian Peninsula and Ethiopia where it originates, is noted for remarkable healing effects on the skin and respiratory tract. Chinese healers used it to treat infected sores and leprosy.

In 1981 some German scientists investigated the "mind-bending" effects of inhaling the aroma and found that a psychoactive substance is produced when the gum is burned. Frankincense also deepens breathing, which can result in calmness, and this could explain how using it as incense creates a state conducive to prayer.

EMOTIONS & MIND

I'll never forget my excitement when, walking in northern Kenya, I came across a frankincense tree and was able to pick off some of the pale yellow resin. Its rich, rejuvenating fragrance helped me to complete that day's hike.

ACHES & PAINS

In India, frankincense has been, and still is, used to treat rheumatic aches.

RESPIRATORY PROBLEMS

Anti-inflammatory, antiseptic, and antifungal. The oil causes the bronchi of the lungs to dilate and may ease the discomfort of lung infections. Once inhaled, it acts upon mucus, enabling sputum to be expelled from the body. Use diluted oil in a chest massage.

SKIN & BEAUTY

Traditionally, frankincense has been used as a perfume base. An Asian friend perfumes her damp hair with the fragrance of the burnt oil. I add

the oil to face products for its lovely perfume and because it is thought to have rejuvenating properties. Add it to a massage oil or cream for dry or aging skin (see page 80).

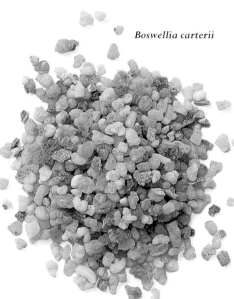

Boswellia carterii

DROPLETS OF GUM RESIN form when the bark of the frankincense tree is scraped. They harden and solidify, then oil is obtained from the resin.

CHEST MASSAGE

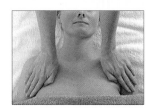

A chest massage with frankincense can deepen breathing (see pages 58–9).

OIL COMBINATIONS

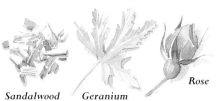

Sandalwood   Geranium   Rose

SANDALWOOD OIL enhances the woody, resinous scent of frankincense oil, while geranium and rose oils sweeten the aroma.

Chamaemelum nobile / Matricaria recutita
CHAMOMILE

One of the gentlest of oils, chamomile has a very soothing effect and is well suited to treating children. It was revered by the Ancient Egyptians and has long been associated with herbal medicine. According to the herbalist Nicholas Culpeper, writing in The English Physician *(1649), "Bathing with a decoction of chamomile taketh away weariness and easeth pain."*

SCENT
Pungent, herbaceous, fruity

NOTE
| MIDDLE |

EXPENSE RATING
✳ ✳ ✳

WARNINGS
See page 16.

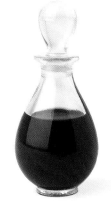

Main constituents:
chamazulene, bisabolol, esters, pinene, linalool

THERAPEUTIC PROPERTIES

This oil is my first choice when needing to calm and soothe. Roman chamomile (*Chamaemelum nobile*) has a high ester content, making it especially soothing. The deep blue color of the oil of German chamomile (*Matricaria recutita*) comes from its high level of chamazulene, which boosts its anti-inflammatory effect. Chamomile is grown in temperate parts of Europe and Eurasia, Egypt, and the U.S.

—— EMOTIONS & MIND ——

Use in massage blends to ease anxiety, insomnia, stress-related headaches, and premenstrual tension.

—— ACHES & PAINS ——

Soothes muscular aches, sprains, and swollen joints (see pages 100–1).

—— DIGESTIVE PROBLEMS ——

Anti-spasmodic. Use to treat colic, flatulence, and indigestion. Massage the abdomen gently with diluted oil.

—— SKIN & BEAUTY ——

Suitable for all skin types. Antiseptic; has healing properties when applied diluted to inflamed skin or abrasions. Excellent remedy for acne, eczema, psoriasis (see pages 108–9), and allergies, rashes, and chapped nipples.

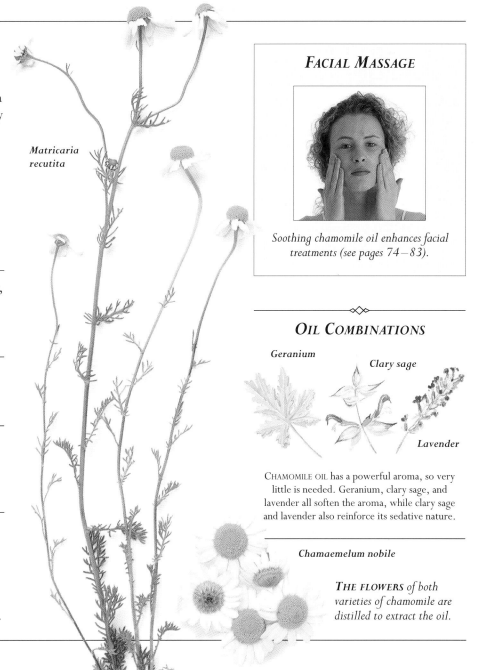

Matricaria recutita

FACIAL MASSAGE

Soothing chamomile oil enhances facial treatments (see pages 74–83).

OIL COMBINATIONS

Geranium

Clary sage

Lavender

CHAMOMILE OIL has a powerful aroma, so very little is needed. Geranium, clary sage, and lavender all soften the aroma, while clary sage and lavender also reinforce its sedative nature.

Chamaemelum nobile

THE FLOWERS *of both varieties of chamomile are distilled to extract the oil.*

Citrus aurantium / Citrus bigaradia / Citrus vulgaris
ORANGE, NEROLI & PETITGRAIN

Native to Asia, the bitter, or Seville, orange tree is thought to have been introduced to Europe along Arab trade routes around AD1200. The tree gained popularity in Spain under Moorish rule, but since oranges were scarce and expensive, they were not often used in European herbal medicine until the late 17th century. By the 18th century, they were being recommended for a great variety of complaints, ranging from melancholia to heart problems and colic. The tree yields three essential citrus oils: orange, neroli, and petitgrain. Today all are used to calm the nerves and combat insomnia.

Citrus aurantium, Citrus bigaradia, Citrus vulgaris

ORANGE

THERAPEUTIC PROPERTIES
Historically, this citrus oil was used in Europe as a mild tonic to treat the nerves, bronchitis, and digestive problems, as it still is in traditional Chinese medicine.

EMOTIONS & MIND
Orange is considered a general tonic. The uplifting, familiar scent can allay anxiety and is popular with children.

DIGESTIVE PROBLEMS
Its anti-spasmodic action helps reduce colic and heartburn. To treat constipation and indigestion, massage the abdomen with diluted oil.

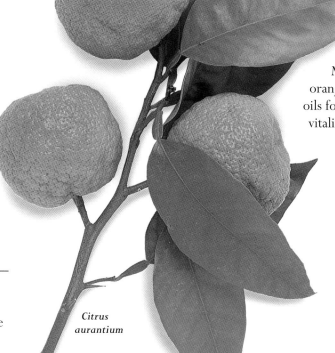

Citrus aurantium

ORANGE OIL is expressed from the rind of the bitter orange fruit.

SKIN & BEAUTY
Mildly astringent. Use orange oil in facial creams or oils for facial massage to bring vitality to the skin.

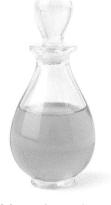

Main constituents: limonene, myrcene, citral, citronellal

SCENT
Fresh, citrus, dry

NOTE		
BASE	MIDDLE	TOP

EXPENSE RATING
*

WARNINGS
Avoid sun & sunlamps for 6 hours; can cause allergies. See page 16.

BACK MASSAGE

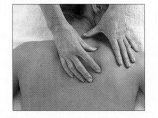

Orange oil, like neroli and petitgrain, can ease stress in the back (see pages 48–53).

OIL COMBINATIONS

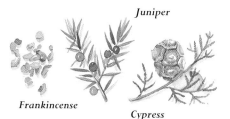

Juniper

Frankincense

Cypress

FRANKINCENSE AND JUNIPER add spice to orange oil, and cypress provides a clean, fresh scent.

Citrus aurantium, Citrus bigaradia

NEROLI

THERAPEUTIC PROPERTIES
One of the most exquisite scents, neroli is prized for its gentle sedative nature. The oil is said to be named after the wife of the Italian prince of Nerola, who used it extensively.

——— EMOTIONS & MIND ———
Extremely beneficial in treating panic attacks and insomnia (see pages 98–9).

——— DIGESTIVE PROBLEMS ———
For stress-related disturbances, such as irritable bowel syndrome, gently massage the abdomen with diluted oil.

——— SKIN & BEAUTY ———
Valuable in skin-care preparations, particularly for mature or sensitive skin and for broken capillaries.

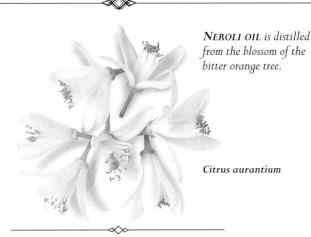

NEROLI OIL is distilled from the blossom of the bitter orange tree.

Citrus aurantium

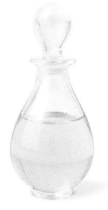

OIL COMBINATIONS

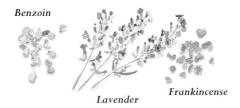

Benzoin

Lavender

Frankincense

BENZOIN AND FRANKINCENSE deepen the scent of neroli and lavender enhances its sedative qualities.

Main constituents: *linalool, limonene, linalyl acetate, nerol, geraniol*

SCENT
Intensely sweet, rich, floral

NOTE		
BASE	MIDDLE	TOP

EXPENSE RATING
✴ ✴ ✴ ✴

WARNINGS
See page 16.

Citrus aurantium

PETITGRAIN

THERAPEUTIC PROPERTIES
Petitgrain oil resembles neroli therapeutically and is also good for nervous and stress-related conditions, including insomnia and jet lag. Both are frequently used in high-quality perfume. Being cheaper and less intense in aroma than neroli, it is also popular in massage oils.

——— EMOTIONS & MIND ———
I use petitgrain for its ability to relieve stress. It is lovely in a bath oil to banish fatigue and relieve anxiety.

——— SKIN & BEAUTY ———
Especially good for irritated skin and acne. Use it in a facial massage or add to homemade face creams (see page 72). It also makes a good hair tonic — add 12 drops to the final rinse.

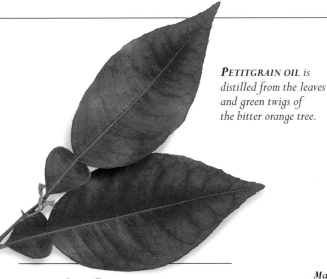

PETITGRAIN OIL is distilled from the leaves and green twigs of the bitter orange tree.

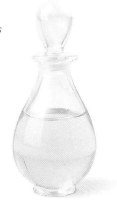

OIL COMBINATIONS

Rosemary

Clary sage

Geranium

GERANIUM OIL rounds out the aroma of petitgrain, while rosemary oil adds sharpness, and clary sage enhances its sedative effects.

Main constituents: *linalyl acetate, linalool, limonene, geraniol, terpineol*

SCENT
Floral, citrus, woody

NOTE		
BASE	MIDDLE	TOP

EXPENSE RATING
✴

WARNINGS
See page 16.

Citrus bergamia
BERGAMOT

Widely used in Italian folk medicine, bergamot takes its name from an Italian village, and its traditional uses include reducing fevers. The delightful perfume is an important ingredient in eau de cologne, and the citrus oil is used to flavor Earl Grey tea. Bergamot oil has an uplifting effect that seems to help allay depression, and nearly everyone likes its fresh, citrusy aroma.

SCENT
Fresh, lively, citrusy

NOTE
BASE   MIDDLE   TOP

EXPENSE RATING
✳ ✳

WARNINGS
Use low dilutions (1%); avoid sun & sunlamps for 6 hours. See page 16.

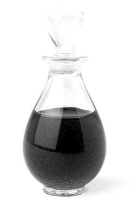

Main constituents: linalyl acetate, limonene, linalool, bergaptene

THERAPEUTIC PROPERTIES

The oil from bergamot, which is cultivated in Italy, South America, and West Africa, lifts the spirits and helps heal wounds and skin problems. Through his research in the 1960s and 70s, the Italian doctor, Paolo Rosvesti, confirmed that bergamot helps relieve depressive states and anxiety. Indian research also found that it helps regulate the appetite.

Its delightful scent makes bergamot popular as an air freshener, with the added benefit that its antiseptic and antiviral properties may protect against airborne bacteria. I burn the oil in a vaporizer in the classroom to help new students feel at ease.

Bergaptene, one of the constituents of the oil, can cause photosensitivity, so wait at least six hours after use before exposing yourself to the sun or a sunlamp (and preferably, wash first). A bergaptene-free oil is also available.

— EMOTIONS & MIND —

Noted for its excellent calming and antidepressant qualities, which are due to a high ester content. Like most citrus oils, bergamot helps improve moods and lift depression. Seems to allay anxiety and grief, especially when used in conjunction with a relaxing face or back massage.

— URINARY PROBLEMS —

Antiseptic. Add well-diluted oil (1%) to the bath to treat urinary cystitis.

— SKIN & BEAUTY —

Its antiseptic properties make bergamot useful in the treatment of acne. Gently stroke the face to

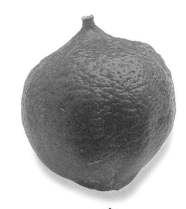

THE OIL *is expressed from the peel of the fruit when nearly ripe but still green.*

stimulate the circulation and lymphatic flow. Bergamot oil's delightful, fresh scent may help alleviate the stress suffered by those with skin problems. The famous French herbalist Maurice Mességué, writing in 1975, recommended it as an excellent disinfectant for wounds, abscesses, and boils (see pages 102–3). Bergamot may cause skin irritation, so use it in low dilutions of 1% or less; never apply it neat.

OIL COMBINATIONS

Juniper

Neroli

Chamomile

BERGAMOT OIL blends with juniper to reinforce its use as an air purifier. Chamomile oil enhances its calming effect, and neroli oil adds depth to the refreshing citrusy perfume.

FACIAL MASSAGE

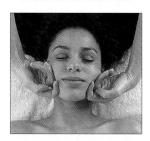

The uplifting effect of bergamot oil enhances facials (see pages 74–9).

Cupressus sempervirens
CYPRESS

*I*n many cultures, the cypress tree has represented eternal life, and Plato (c.429 – 47BC) referred to it as the symbol of immortality. The oil has a fresh, spicy aroma that many people find refreshing, and in Ancient Greece it was customary to send tuberculosis patients into a cypress grove to breathe the air and ease their symptoms. Cypress oil is still used to treat respiratory complaints.

SCENT
Spicy, sweet, balsamic, refreshing

NOTE
BASE   MIDDLE   TOP

EXPENSE RATING
*

WARNINGS
Avoid in the first three months of pregnancy. See page 16.

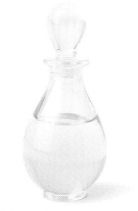

Main constituents: *pinene, carene, myrcene, camphene, sylvestrene*

THERAPEUTIC PROPERTIES

Cypress was burned as incense in the ancient world for purification, and was used because of its anti-spasmodic properties to treat respiratory problems. In traditional Chinese and Indian Ayurvedic medicine, it was recognized for its astringent effects.

In 1597 John Gerard, herbalist to King James I of England, wrote in *The Herball or Generall Historie of Plantes* that "the leaves and nuts are good to cure the rupture," and today the oil is used to treat hemorrhoids, varicose veins, broken capillaries, and bruising. Since the 16th century, cypress has been advocated as an insect repellent. Gerard also advised people to "use the smoke of the leaves to drive away gnats…and the wood laid amongst garments preserveth against the moths."

—*ACHES & PAINS* —
I have found it useful in massage blends to treat rheumatic aches; or in a cold compress, when massage is inadvisable – for example, in reducing the spread of recent bruising or on varicose veins or when rheumatic joints are inflamed.

FOOT MASSAGE

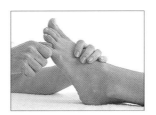

Cypress oil helps inhibit sweat and refresh the feet (see pages 66–7).

OIL COMBINATIONS

Citrus oils   *Frankincense*
               Rose

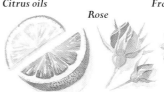

CYPRESS OIL blends well with all citrus oils in tonics and with rose oil for facial massage blends, while frankincense brings out the incenselike nature of the aroma.

THE NEEDLES and twigs of the tree are distilled to extract the oil.

— *RESPIRATORY PROBLEMS* —
Anti-spasmodic. Eases coughs, asthma, bronchitis, and sore throats. Put a couple of drops on a handkerchief and inhale deeply.

——— *SKIN & BEAUTY* ———
Astringent; good for oily skin. I find the aroma of cypress oil appeals particularly to men. Use in facial steaming, skin tonics, or aftershaves. Often included in anti-cellulite blends (see pages 106–7). Helpful for people who suffer from sweaty feet. Add a couple of drops to a daily foot bath, or massage the feet with diluted oil.

Cymbopogon citratus
LEMONGRASS

A traditional ingredient in Malaysian and Thai cooking, lemongrass is also the source of an essential oil that has valuable therapeutic uses. In addition to acting as a digestive tonic, diuretic and antiseptic, the oil has pain-relieving properties. Combined with massage, the powerful lemony aroma makes a great restorative for physical and emotional problems. Men especially like its strong, fresh scent.

SCENT
Lemony, grasslike, dry, fresh

NOTE

BASE	MIDDLE	TOP

EXPENSE RATING
*

WARNINGS
Possible skin irritation, use low dilutions (1%). See page 16.

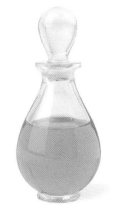

Main constituents: citral, linalool, geraniol, myrcene, citronellal

THERAPEUTIC PROPERTIES
Lemongrass is considered a cooling herb in India, and citral, its major constituent, has sedative and anti-septic effects. In India, it is used widely in Ayurvedic medicine to treat fevers and infections, and recent research here has confirmed the oil's analgesic and anti-fungal properties and its ability to reduce fevers. Use with caution on the face, neck, and delicate skin. Lemongrass is cultivated in Africa, Asia, and the West Indies.

EMOTIONS & MIND
Acts as a sedative on the central nervous system. Use to counteract mental fatigue (see pages 98–9).

ACHES & PAINS
I use well-diluted lemongrass oil to massage athletes after sports, especially if they are drained of energy.

DIGESTIVE PROBLEMS
Considered to be a tonic for the digestive system. Massage a well-diluted oil blend into the abdomen.

SKIN & BEAUTY
Antiseptic. Lemongrass oil is used for treating acne (see pages 108–9).

ABDOMEN MASSAGE

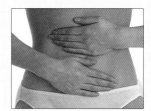

Use lemongrass in a massage oil blend as a tonic for the digestion (see page 88).

OIL COMBINATIONS

Sandalwood

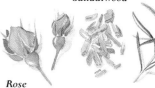

Rose

Rosemary

LEMONGRASS OIL blends well with rose and sandalwood oils, which soften its strong aroma, and with rosemary oil, which enhances its refreshing scent.

LEMONGRASS essential oil is extracted from the grass by the process of steam distillation.

Eucalyptus globulus
EUCALYPTUS

*E*asily recognized by its camphorlike vapor, eucalyptus is the classic remedy for respiratory problems and is contained in many commercial products for colds and nasal congestion. It is also used for chest complaints, musculoskeletal problems, and to purify the air. Originally from Australia, the tree was introduced to Europe in the late 18th century and distilled commercially in the 1850s.

SCENT
Camphorlike, sweet, woody

NOTE
BASE MIDDLE **TOP**

EXPENSE RATING
*

WARNINGS
Use low dilutions (1%); avoid with homeopathic remedies. See page 16.

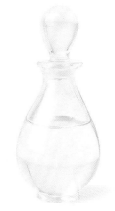

Main constituents: cineol, pinene, limonene

THERAPEUTIC PROPERTIES

Traditionally, Australian Aboriginal peoples bound the leaves of the indigenous eucalyptus tree to wounds to speed healing. Recent research has confirmed the oil's pain-relieving and anti-inflammatory properties, and its ability to reduce swelling and accelerate healing.

ACHES & PAINS

Eucalyptus oil feels cool to the skin but warm to the muscles. The cineol content makes it analgesic, and it also reduces fevers (see pages 100–1).

RESPIRATORY PROBLEMS

The main constituent of eucalyptus essential oil, cineol, is responsible for its powerful antiseptic, antiviral, and expectorant effects. Use in a steam inhalation (see pages 102–3), put two drops on a handkerchief and inhale, or massage the chest with diluted oil.

ALLERGIES & INFECTIONS

It has antibacterial properties, is a good antiviral agent and stimulates the immune system. When used in a vaporizer, the essential oil reduces airborne microbes.

OIL COMBINATIONS

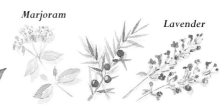

Marjoram

Lavender

Juniper

MARJORAM OIL boosts the decongestant effect of eucalyptus oil, juniper oil adds a clean scent, and lavender softens the aroma and enhances the harmony of the blend.

CHEST MASSAGE

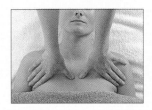

The powerful scent relaxes the chest and can ease congestion (see pages 58–9).

THE LEAVES of the plant, cultivated in Australia and southern Europe, are distilled to extract the oil.

Jasminum officinale / Jasminum grandiflorum
JASMINE

*E*xquisitely fragranced, jasmine is reputed to be an aphrodisiac. In the 16th century, the Grand Duke of Tuscany procured a plant from India. Determined to keep it to himself, he forbade his gardener to give cuttings away. Yet the gardener gave his beloved a posy containing jasmine. Delighted by its aroma, she planted the jasmine, sold cuttings, and saved enough money to wed the poor gardener.

SCENT
Sweet, heady, rich, floral

NOTE
BASE | MIDDLE | TOP

EXPENSE RATING
✳ ✳ ✳ ✳

WARNINGS
Avoid in pregnancy and on babies.
Can cause headaches. See page 16.

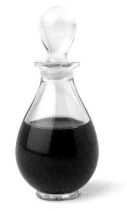

Main constituents: benzyl acetate, linalool, linalyl acetate, jasmone

THERAPEUTIC PROPERTIES

The flowers of the jasmine plant, which is cultivated in India and North Africa, yield tiny amounts of oil, making it very expensive. It is valued in the Far East and the Indian subcontinent for its medicinal properties and scent. In China, the flowers have been used to treat dysentery and hepatitis. In Indian Ayurvedic medicine, jasmine is recommended for cleansing the blood.

Garlands of jasmine are presented to honored guests in India, and in some areas, ten days before marriage, brides are massaged daily with *Ubtan*, a blend of herbs, spices, jasmine, and sweet almond oil that cleanses and smooths the skin and scents it with the heady aroma of jasmine.

EMOTIONS & MIND

Uplifting and stimulating. I believe the heavenly aroma acts as an anti-depressant. Use to treat lethargy (see pages 98–9).

GYNECOLOGICAL PROBLEMS

In India, the flowers are traditionally applied to the breasts to suppress excess lactation after childbirth. For menstrual cramps, massage the lower back and abdomen with diluted oil.

Jasminum officinale

THE STAR-SHAPED flowers are picked at night, and oil is extracted using solvent.

SKIN & BEAUTY

Jasmine oil is frequently used in skin-care preparations for its delicious perfume and invigorating effect (see page 75).

SCALP MASSAGE

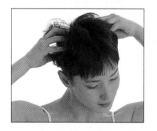

Use jasmine oil in a refreshing massage to perfume the scalp (see page 85).

OIL COMBINATIONS

Clary sage *Sandalwood* *Citrus oils*

CLARY SAGE emphasizes the sensual aspect of the oil. In India, jasmine oil is traditionally blended with exotic sandalwood oil, while citrus oils freshen its aroma.

Juniperus communis
JUNIPER

*R*enowned for its cleansing properties, juniper has been used through the ages to purify body, mind, and spirit. It has been valued by all the great civilizations since Ancient Egypt to fight infection and for purification ceremonies (sprigs with berries were said to keep witches away). Its antiviral properties make juniper useful in treating respiratory infections and an ideal air freshener.

SCENT
Woody, fresh, sweet

NOTE
BASE	MIDDLE	TOP

EXPENSE RATING
✻

WARNINGS
Avoid in pregnancy, kidney disease, or glomerulonephritis. See page 16.

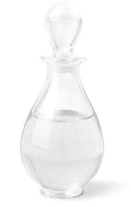

Main constituents: pinene, myrcene, limonene

THERAPEUTIC PROPERTIES

In Ancient Greece, juniper was burned as incense to combat epidemics, as it was in a cholera outbreak in Germany in 1856, and a smallpox epidemic in France in 1870. Cato the Elder (234–149BC), a Roman, considered the berries to be diuretic, as did Gerard, who wrote that "it provoketh urine." Culpeper said the plant "provokes urine exceedingly…helps the gout and sciatica, and strengthens the limbs of the body." Juniper oil is still used in similar ways.

——— EMOTIONS & MIND ———
Calming and fresh. Use diluted in a bath or massage oil to ease stress.

——— ACHES & PAINS ———
Diuretic and local stimulant, useful for rheumatic problems and sports aches and pains. The constituent myrcene has analgesic properties. Dilute with a carrier oil and blend with rosemary oil for use in the bath or with ginger oil for massage (see pages 100–1).

——— SKIN & BEAUTY ———
Antiseptic; use in toners and men's aftershaves. Useful for treating acne; apply a cold compress or diluted oil. Helpful in a massage used to aid slimming or combat cellulite.

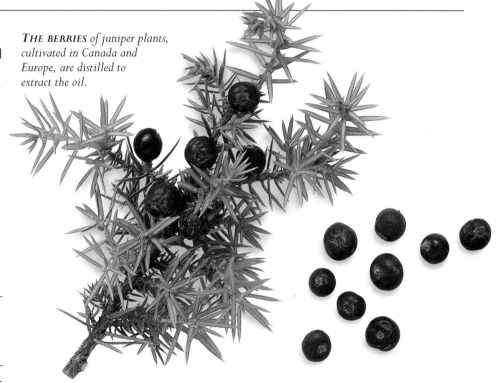

THE BERRIES of juniper plants, cultivated in Canada and Europe, are distilled to extract the oil.

THIGH MASSAGE

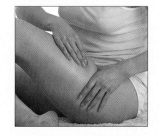

Juniper oil is often used in anti-cellulite massage blends (see pages 88–9).

OIL COMBINATIONS

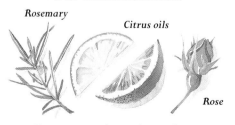

Rosemary

Citrus oils

Rose

ROSEMARY OIL enhances the stimulating, rubefacient (skin-reddening) effect of juniper oil, citrus oils complement its calming properties, and rose oil sweetens its scent.

Lavandula angustifolia / Lavandula officinalis
LAVENDER

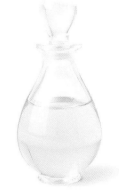

*L*avender is probably the most versatile and widely used essential oil. Deriving its name from the Latin lavare, *to wash, it may have been used by the Romans in bathwater. Due to its sedative nature, lavender has long been recommended as a folk remedy for insomnia — for example, in herbal pillows. Recently it has been employed in many hospitals to help patients relax and sleep better.*

SCENT
Sweet, floral, herbaceous, stimulating, piercing

NOTE
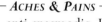
BASE   MIDDLE   TOP

EXPENSE RATING
✳

WARNINGS
See page 16.

Main constituents: *linalyl acetate, linalool, caryophyllene, lavandulyl acetate, cineol, geraniol*

THERAPEUTIC PROPERTIES

Lavender is used primarily for its sedative and antiseptic properties. *Lavandula officinalis* and *L. angustifolia* are known as true lavender and yield the finest oil, while *L. latifolia* and *L. fragrans* hybrids yield more oil, albeit with less sedative properties. In 1910, Réné Maurice Gattefossé, a French perfumer and chemist, rinsed his hands in lavender essence, thereby halting the onset of gangrene that had developed from a burn. His swift and successful recovery was a catalyst for research into the properties of essential oils.

THE FLOWERING *tops are distilled to extract the oil.*

Lavandula angustifolia

EMOTIONS & MIND
Sedative and calming, lavender is the perfect oil to treat insomnia. Use in a massage blend or diluted in the bath, or put a drop on your pillow.

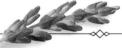

OIL COMBINATIONS

Marjoram   **Citrus oils**   **Frankincense**

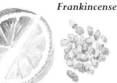

MARJORAM enhances lavender's sedative effect, citrus oils increase its floral quality, and frankincense heightens its soothing and expectorant properties.

ACHES & PAINS
Analgesic, anti-spasmodic. Use in a massage blend or add diluted oil to the bath to relieve muscular aches and pains. Excellent as a headache remedy; simply massage a little oil slowly and gently around the temples.

RESPIRATORY PROBLEMS
Inhale to speed recovery from colds, bronchitis, influenza, and throat infections. Use in a stimulating chest massage to relieve congestion.

SKIN & BEAUTY
Antiseptic; use to treat acne and eczema (see pages 108–9), to soothe insect bites and stings, to clean and disinfect cuts and sores, and to help heal minor burns (see pages 102–3).

BACK MASSAGE

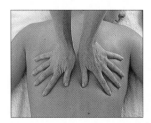

A soporific massage with lavender oil can help induce sleep (see pages 48–53).

Melaleuca alternifolia
TEA TREE

This species of paperbark tree, native to the sub-tropical coast of New South Wales and parts of Queensland, Australia, has a long history of use as a potent antiseptic. Aboriginal peoples used poultices of the leaves on wounds and cuts, and smoked the leaves to clear congestion. Tea tree oil remains one of aromatherapy's most powerful tools in the fight against bacteria, fungi, yeast, and viruses.

SCENT
Medicinal, spicy, fresh

NOTE

BASE	MIDDLE	TOP

EXPENSE RATING
✳

WARNINGS
For sensitive skin, use a normal dilution (2½%). See page 16.

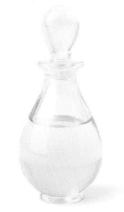

Main constituents: *terpineol, terpinene, cineol, cymene, pinene*

THERAPEUTIC PROPERTIES

The name *tea tree* first appeared in Captain Cook's "Voyage towards the South Pole and around the World 1772–5." Its properties were again recognized in 1923 by Arthur Penfold, a New South Wales chemist, and several papers were published in the 1930s describing its use as an antiseptic with varied uses and very low toxicity. During World War II, Australian soldiers were issued the oil, but its use declined with the advent of antibiotics after the war. From the 1970s it became popular again. Often referred to as the first-aid kit in a bottle, tea tree oil is invaluable for treating minor wounds, infections, cuts, stings, and acne.

— RESPIRATORY PROBLEMS —
To relieve sore throats, coughs, nasal and chest congestion, place a couple of drops of tea tree oil on a handkerchief and inhale.

— GYNECOLOGICAL PROBLEMS —
Add diluted oil to the bath to treat urinary cystitis or *Candida albicans,* which causes yeast infections.

— SKIN & BEAUTY —
For acne, dab undiluted oil on isolated pimples 1–2 times a day, or use

THE ESSENTIAL OIL is extracted from the leaves using steam distillation.

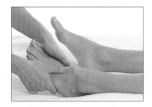

diluted in a skin tonic. To soothe insect bites, stings, cuts, wounds, and cold sores, apply oil undiluted. To combat athlete's foot, corns, calluses, or smelly feet, add 5–10 drops to a daily footbath. Cool minor burns with cold water, then apply the oil.

FOOT MASSAGE

Tea tree is antiseptic and antifungal and thus ideal for the feet (see pages 66–7).

OIL COMBINATIONS

Geranium   *Lemon*

Scot's pine

TEA TREE is hard to blend, but geranium sweetens its scent, Scot's pine emphasizes its spicy, medicinal aroma, and lemon brings out its freshness.

Melissa officinalis
MELISSA

*T*he delicious scent of melissa (lemon balm) can hardly fail to lift one's spirits. I have a bush by my front door so that whenever I go in or out of the house I can take a few leaves, crush them, and enjoy the effects. It is this uplifting quality of melissa that I find most therapeutic. I use it as an antidepressant oil, especially if a client needs soothing and boosting with a general tonic.

SCENT
Soft, lemony, herbaceous

NOTE

BASE	MIDDLE	TOP

EXPENSE RATING
✿ ✿ ✿ ✿

WARNINGS
Possible skin irritation, so use low dilutions (1%). See page 16.

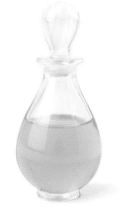

Main constituents: linalool, geraniol, citronellal, citral

THERAPEUTIC PROPERTIES

Refreshing and calming to mind and body, melissa can help those suffering from depression, anxiety, shock, or bereavement. It was used in medieval "elixirs of youth" and according to Culpeper, "It causes the mind and heart to become merry...and driveth away all troublesome cares and thoughts." Cultivated in Europe and the U.S., the essential oil is frequently adulterated; ask your source for melissa "true" instead of melissa "type."

— EMOTIONS & MIND—
Calms, uplifts, revitalizes, and restores emotional balance. Dilute well with a carrier oil and use to massage the whole body, or add a few drops to bathwater.

— DIGESTIVE PROBLEMS —
For digestive complaints that are accompanied by tension or anxiety, gently massage the abdomen with diluted melissa.

— GYNECOLOGICAL PROBLEMS —
Thought to help regulate ovulation and menstruation, especially if irregularity is caused by emotional upset. Apply in a massage oil to the abdomen and lower back.

MELISSA OIL is extracted from the leaves by steam distillation.

— SKIN & BEAUTY —
Antiseptic, antiviral, and antifungal. Relieves skin problems, including cold sores. Apply well diluted.

BACK MASSAGE

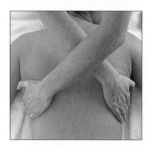

For a soothing effect, use melissa oil in a back massage (see pages 48–53).

OIL COMBINATIONS

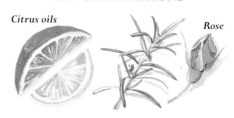

Citrus oils

Rose

Rosemary

MELISSA combines with citrus oils to enhance its sedative qualities and is balanced by the sharpness of rosemary and the luxurious aroma of rose.

Mentha piperita
PEPPERMINT

Refreshing and energizing, peppermint reminds me of Morocco, where it grows in abundance and is served as a delicious tea. Peppermint is an excellent mental stimulant, and as a digestive it is unsurpassed. It also helps alleviate stomach pains. I once used a very weak dilution of oil to massage a baby with colic. The results were immediate: the baby stopped crying and fell asleep.

SCENT
Minty, grasslike, balsamic, fresh

NOTE
BASE **MIDDLE** TOP

EXPENSE RATING
�֍ ✖

WARNINGS
Use low dilutions (1%); avoid with homeopathic remedies. See page 16.

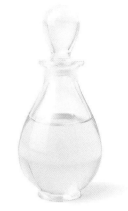

Main constituents: menthol, menthone, cineol

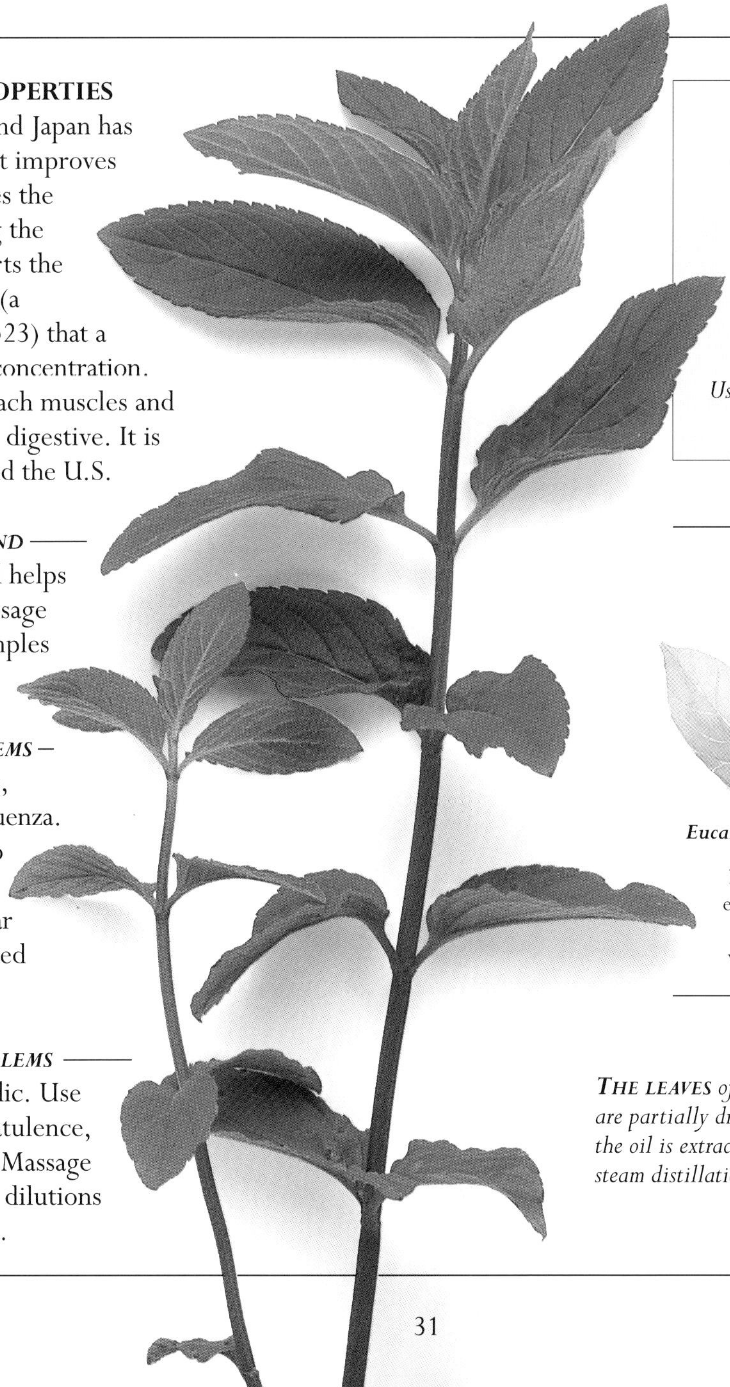

THERAPEUTIC PROPERTIES

Research in the U.S. and Japan has shown that peppermint improves alertness and stimulates the brain without affecting the heart rate. This supports the idea of Pliny the Elder (a Roman writer born AD 23) that a mint crown could aid concentration. Mint soothes the stomach muscles and has long been used as a digestive. It is cultivated in Europe and the U.S.

——EMOTIONS & MIND——
Improves alertness and helps relieve headaches. Massage diluted oil into the temples or add to a bath.

—RESPIRATORY PROBLEMS—
Powerful decongestant, good for colds and influenza. Massage diluted oil into the temples or use steam inhalation to clear nasal passages. Prolonged use can disturb sleep.

——DIGESTIVE PROBLEMS——
Calming, anti-spasmodic. Use peppermint to treat flatulence, indigestion, and colic. Massage the abdomen with low dilutions of oil (see pages 62–3).

FOOT MASSAGE

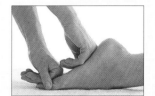

Use peppermint oil in a cooling massage for tired feet (see pages 66–7).

OIL COMBINATIONS

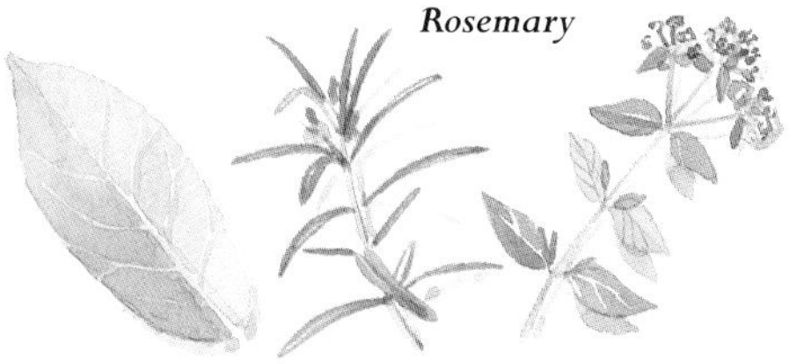

Rosemary

Eucalyptus   Marjoram

PEPPERMINT OIL combines perfectly with eucalyptus and rosemary, which reinforce its effects on colds and influenza, and with warming and penetrating marjoram oil.

THE LEAVES of peppermint are partially dried before the oil is extracted by steam distillation.

Origanum majorana
MARJORAM

A pungent herb from the mint family, marjoram was reputedly created by Aphrodite, the Greek goddess of love, as a symbol of happiness and well-being. If the plant grew on a grave, happiness of the deceased was assured. Marjoram has been known since ancient times as a friend to the nerves and useful to women. I use the oil to calm the mind and ease taut muscles.

SCENT
Camphorlike, sweet, warm

NOTE
BASE	MIDDLE	TOP

EXPENSE RATING
✳ ✳

WARNINGS
Avoid in pregnancy; use low dilutions (1%). See page 16.

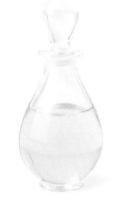

Main constituents: methyl chavicol, terpineol, eugenol, linalool, and many terpenes

THERAPEUTIC PROPERTIES
Gerard and Culpeper credited marjoram with the ability to comfort and warm the brain and benefit stiff, cold joints, and respiratory disorders. It is antiseptic, anti-spasmodic, and antifungal. Japanese research has confirmed its sedative effects. Marjoram is cultivated in central and southern Europe, and Egypt.

EMOTIONS & MIND
To treat insomnia or to restore frayed nerves, use diluted oil in a warm bath or with a soothing back massage to induce a good night's sleep.

ACHES & PAINS
Wonderful for treating rheumatic aches and cold, contracted muscles, and a great antidote to aches and stiffness from overenthusiastic exercise. Apply diluted oil in a massage, a compress, or add to the bath (see pages 100–1).

RESPIRATORY PROBLEMS
One of the best remedies to treat colds and chills. Put a few drops of oil on a handkerchief and inhale to clear sinuses and ease headaches. Use in an inhalation for bronchitis and nasal congestion (see pages 102–3).

GYNECOLOGICAL PROBLEMS
The warming and calming effects of marjoram oil help relieve menstrual cramps. Slowly and rhythmically massage the abdomen and lower back with diluted oil or apply a warm compress to the abdomen.

LEG MASSAGE

Massage with marjoram oil eases aches (see pages 54–5, 64–5).

THE FLOWERS AND LEAVES of marjoram plants are used, and the oil is extracted by steam distillation.

OIL COMBINATIONS

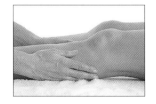

Eucalyptus   *Lavender*

Rosemary

ROSEMARY AND EUCALYPTUS OILS reinforce the benefits of marjoram to ease colds and muscular aches. Lavender enhances its sedative qualities.

Pelargonium graveolens
GERANIUM

*O*riginating in southern Africa, geraniums were brought to Europe in the 17th century. Over 700 species exist, many of them highly perfumed. The scent of geranium oil resembles rose, with which it shares many constituents. Consequently, it is often added to rose oil to extend it. The soothing aroma helps reduce stress and, as so many people love the scent, I use it often in facial treatments.

SCENT
Sweet, round, floral, herbaceous

NOTE

BASE	MIDDLE	TOP

EXPENSE RATING
✳ ✳

WARNINGS
Use low dilutions (1%). See page 16.

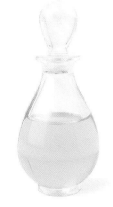

Main constituents: geraniol, linalool, citronellol

THERAPEUTIC PROPERTIES

Traditionally geranium was used to stanch bleeding, heal wounds, ulcers, and skin disorders, and treat diarrhea, dysentery, and colic. Antibacterial properties and insecticidal actions were found when geranium was screened for medicinal usage in a joint project of the laboratories of the Royal Botanic Gardens, Kew, and the Society of Applied Science, in Britain. I use the diluted oil for first aid on minor cuts and burns. Geranium oil is also an effective insect repellent, useful to keep in a first-aid kit.

—— *EMOTIONS & MIND* ——
Antidepressant. Excellent relaxant for those suffering from nervous tension. Use in inhalations, diluted in the bath, or in a massage blend.

—— *GYNECOLOGICAL PROBLEMS* ——
In a French study of 1933, it was found to be active against *Candida albicans*, which causes vaginal yeast infections. Also used to regulate premenstrual mood swings (see pages 106–7).

—— *SKIN & BEAUTY* ——
Rich in the gentle alcohols geraniol and linalool, it is suitable for all skin. Good for acne treatments because of

its antimicrobial effect. Add to massage blends for the face, to skin toners, and creams (see pages 70–3). Popular in anti-cellulite massage blends to relieve fluid retention: gently massage the affected area.

GERANIUM OIL is extracted by steam distillation of the whole plant. It is cultivated in Egypt, Russia, and the French island of Réunion.

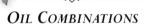

OIL COMBINATIONS

Juniper

Chamomile

Citrus oils

CHAMOMILE, JUNIPER, AND CITRUS OILS mellow the sweet-scented oil. Chamomile also enhances its effectiveness against cuts or inflammation.

HAND MASSAGE

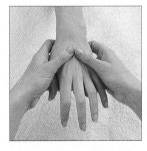

The floral aroma of geranium oil leaves hands lightly fragranced (see pages 60–1).

Rosa centifolia / Rosa damascena
ROSE

*A*ccording to legend, rose oil was discovered at the wedding feast of the Mogul princess Noor Jehan. Rosewater poured into a canal encircling the garden separated in the sun's heat, and the bridal couple gathered the droplets of aromatic oil. Since antiquity, the healing virtues of rose oil have been celebrated, but its exquisite scent still cannot be imitated: it has about 300 constituents, not all known.

SCENT
Intense, lingering, floral

NOTE
BASE   MIDDLE   TOP

EXPENSE RATING
✳ ✳ ✳ ✳

WARNINGS
See page 16.

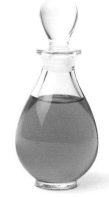

Main constituents: citronellol, geraniol, nerol, linalool, citral, eugenol, phenyl ethanol

THERAPEUTIC PROPERTIES

Roses have long been associated with Venus, Roman goddess of love and beauty, and the oil is still used in beauty products. Avicenna, a philosopher and physician from Bukhara (born AD 980), claimed that rose oil quickened the mind. Since the oil yield from roses is low, it is very costly. For therapeutic use, oil distilled without heat, "phytol," or by steam, "attar," is best; oil extracted by solvent, "absolute," is less pure.

EMOTIONS & MIND
Antidepressant. A 1969 Bulgarian study found that rose oil increases alertness and gives pleasant dreams.

OIL COMBINATIONS

Sandalwood

Lavender

Chamomile

THE BEAUTIFUL, PIERCING SCENT OF ROSE combines perfectly with lavender and chamomile, which bring out its freshness. Sandalwood makes it deeper and more exotic.

Rosa centifolia

THE FLOWERS are the source of the oil: 440 lb (200 kg) of petals produce about 1¾ pints (1 liter) of rose attar. Most roses come from Bulgaria, France, Morocco, Turkey, and Russia.

DIGESTIVE PROBLEMS
In Bulgaria it is used as a liver tonic; in China, as a cure for liver stagnation. Eases hangovers (see pages 104–5).

GYNECOLOGICAL PROBLEMS
A soothing, relaxing massage with rose oil helps ease premenstrual tension.

SKIN & BEAUTY
Antihistamine, antiseptic. Use in facial massage and skin products to calm and uplift (see page 75). A rosewater compress can ease signs of stress in the face by relieving eye strain, headaches, and inflammation.

FACIAL MASSAGE

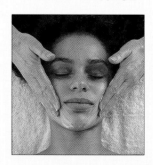

Soothing rose oil has a cooling effect on the face (see pages 74–9).

Rosmarinus officinalis
ROSEMARY

*R*evered as the herb sacred to remembrance, rosemary was said by Culpeper to "help a weak memory and quicken the senses." In medieval times, it was strewn on the floor and carried in nosegays to inhale in oppressive conditions. The herb was thought to ward off evil spirits and to be an elixir of youth and life. I often use rosemary in skin toners for its refreshing and invigorating qualities.

SCENT
Piercing, fresh, herbaceous

NOTE
| BASE | MIDDLE | TOP |

EXPENSE RATING
✳

WARNINGS
Avoid in pregnancy, high blood pressure, and epilepsy. See page 16.

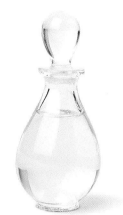

Main constituents: pinene, cineol, camphor, camphene, bornyl acetate, borneol

THERAPEUTIC PROPERTIES

Traditionally rosemary was used as a fumigant for sickrooms and to protect against infectious disease. It was also known for its invigorating, uplifting qualities. Research in 1987 found that the herb has a stimulating effect on the central nervous system, which supports similar claims made by Shakespeare, Culpeper, and Gerard.

EMOTIONS & MIND
Invigorating and stimulating. Use for massaging the face and head (see page 98–9).

ACHES & PAINS
Stimulates the skin to boost circulation and ease pain. For rheumatic aches, use in massage oil; if joint is inflamed, omit massage and use a compress instead (see pages 100–1).

RESPIRATORY PROBLEMS
The scent eases cold symptoms and clears congestion. Put two drops on a handkerchief and inhale or massage the chest with diluted oil.

FRESH FLOWERING tops from Mediterranean countries are used to make top-quality oil.

LEG MASSAGE

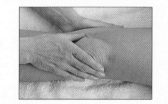

The stimulating action of rosemary oil eases aches (see pages 64–5).

DIGESTIVE PROBLEMS
Relieves headaches that are related to indigestion (see pages 104–5).

ALLERGIES & INFECTIONS
Antifungal, antibacterial. Use as a disinfectant to help prevent infection and deodorize the air (see page 97).

SKIN & BEAUTY
Has a refreshing, invigorating effect on the skin and is effective in toners (see page 72). After washing hair, add to the final rinse to stimulate the scalp, clear dandruff, and increase shine.

OIL COMBINATIONS
Juniper

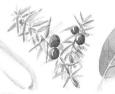

Lemongrass

Petitgrain

THE HEALING PROPERTIES OF ROSEMARY are enhanced when blended with lemongrass and juniper for muscular aches. Lemongrass and petitgrain, like all citrus-scented oils, soften the aroma.

Salvia sclarea
CLARY SAGE

To the Romans, clary sage was a cure-all; the Latin name means "to save." I grow this beautiful herb in my garden, and it gives off a sweet, heady aroma that some people find intoxicating. I often use the essential oil on clients who are convalescing after being in the hospital — it is a powerful relaxant with a warm aroma that promotes sleep and a sense of well-being.

SCENT
Warm, nutty, herbaceous

NOTE

BASE	MIDDLE	TOP

EXPENSE RATING
✳ ✳

WARNINGS
Avoid in pregnancy; may cause vivid dreams; avoid alcohol. See page 16.

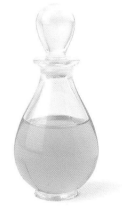

Main constituents: *linalyl acetate, linalool, pinene, myrcene, sclareol*

THERAPEUTIC PROPERTIES
This plant, cultivated in France and Russia, does not share the potential toxicity of sage. Both Culpeper and Gerard commented on its use as a remedy for inflammation and its ability to bring on menstruation. The oil should be avoided in pregnancy, however, until labor. These properties were confirmed in 1938 by biologists who recommended it for aches and pains associated with menstruation. Clary sage is an extremely potent sedative, but in high doses it can leave one feeling almost stupefied.

EMOTIONS & MIND
Promotes sleep; its euphoric effects are often reflected in an immense sense of well-being. To treat depression or nervous exhaustion, use diluted oil in a slow, soporific back massage or in the bath.

RESPIRATORY PROBLEMS
To ease sore throats, put a couple of drops on a handkerchief and inhale.

GYNECOLOGICAL PROBLEMS
Anti-spasmodic, warming, analgesic. Good for relieving menstrual cramps: use in a warm compress (see pages 106–7) or a gentle abdomen massage.

CLARY SAGE OIL *is extracted through steam distillation of the leaves and flowering tops of the plant.*

SKIN & BEAUTY
Widely used in perfumery. The nutty aroma appeals to men and blends with other warm scents. Use in toners and massage oils (see pages 71–2).

ABDOMEN MASSAGE

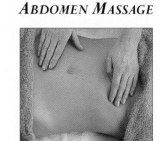

The anti-spasmodic properties of clary sage relieve cramps (see pages 62–3).

OIL COMBINATIONS

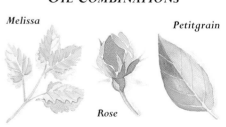

Melissa

Petitgrain

Rose

MELISSA AND PETITGRAIN enhance the sedative, powerfully relaxing properties of clary sage oil, while rose oil strengthens its uplifting, antidepressant quality.

Santalum album
SANDALWOOD

*M*entioned in the Nirkuta, *the oldest of the Hindu Vedas (written in the 5th century* BC), *sandalwood was used in religious ceremonies and plays a key role in Indian Ayurvedic medicine. It is widely used in perfumery for its base note and classic Oriental scent. It is one of my favorite oils; nearly everyone loves its warm, exotic perfume, and I use it to sedate and pamper my clients.*

SCENT
Sweet, woody, balsamic

NOTE
BASE MIDDLE TOP

EXPENSE RATING
✳ ✳ ✳

WARNINGS
See page 16.

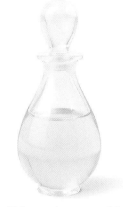

Main constituent: santalol

THERAPEUTIC PROPERTIES

Sandalwood is used to calm and cool the body, reduce inflammation, infection and fever, and to ease sunstroke. I was introduced to it when traveling in India, where 70% of the world's supply is grown (the best oil comes from the Mysore district in southern India). An Indian doctor recommended it as the perfect oil for balancing the skin – he used it to soothe inflammation and to calm sensitive, dry, dehydrated skin.

On the last day of the year, it was customary for Burmese women to sprinkle a mixture of sandalwood oil and rosewater on those nearby, to wash away the year's sins and purify the body and spirit.

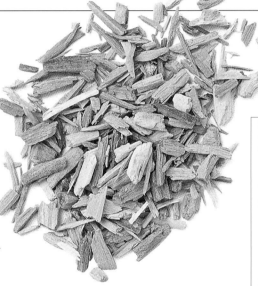

THE HEARTWOOD *of the tree trunk is used, and the oil is extracted from it by steam distillation.*

FACIAL MASSAGE

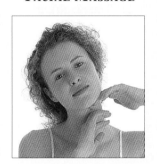

Add sandalwood oil to a pampering massage blend (see pages 80–3).

EMOTIONS & MIND

Calming to the mind and emotions; sedative. It enhances the sense of peace that occurs during meditation. Use in massage blends or in a vaporizer (see page 97) to treat anxiety and depression.

RESPIRATORY PROBLEMS

Sandalwood oil is used to treat laryngitis, sore throats, bronchitis, and chest tightness. Put a couple of drops on a handkerchief and inhale, or massage the area with diluted oil.

URINARY PROBLEMS

Gently antiseptic and diuretic. To treat urinary cystitis, use in a warm compress or bath, or massage diluted oil over the lower back.

ALLERGIES & INFECTIONS

In a French study carried out in 1993, santalol – sandalwood oil's main constituent – was found to be effective in helping treat gonorrhea.

SKIN & BEAUTY

Soothing, anti-inflammatory. The oil is beneficial to acne, eczema, and chapped, dry skin (see pages 108–9) and is popular in beauty products for its sweet, long-lasting fragrance.

OIL COMBINATIONS

Jasmine

Frankincense

Rose

IN INDIA, SANDALWOOD is blended with jasmine and frankincense to increase its exotic aroma and with rose to help create a harmonious scent.

OTHER USEFUL ESSENTIAL OILS

ESSENTIAL OIL	SCENT	NOTE	EXPENSE RATING	SOURCE & EXTRACTION
Styrax benzoin **BENZOIN**	*Sweet, balsamic, warm, like vanilla*	Base: strong Middle: strong Top: mild	✳	Oil is extracted from the gum using solvent. Cultivated in Southeast Asia.
Piper nigrum **BLACK PEPPER**	*Warm, spicy, peppery*	Base: weak Middle: strong Top: strong	✳ ✳	Oil is extracted from the berries (dried peppercorns) by steam distillation. Cultivated in India, Sri Lanka, Indonesia, Malaysia.
Cedrus atlantica **CEDARWOOD**	*Woody – like a freshly sharpened pencil*	Base: strong Middle: strong Top: weak	✳	Oil is extracted from the wood by steam distillation. Cultivated in the Atlas Mountains of Morocco.
Zingiber officinale **GINGER**	*Spicy, fresh, camphory*	Base: strong Middle: strong Top: mild	✳	Oil is extracted from dried, unpeeled rhizome by steam distillation. Cultivated in China and India.
Citrus limonum **LEMON**	*Refreshing, clean, lively*	Base: weak Middle: weak Top: strong	✳	Oil is expressed from the peel of fruit. Cultivated in the Mediterranean and North America.
Citrus reticulata **MANDARIN**	*Light, fresh, fruity, popular with children and older people*	Base: weak Middle: weak Top: strong	✳	Oil is expressed from the peel of fruit. Cultivated in the Mediterranean, Middle East, Europe, and North and South America.
Pogostemon patchouli **PATCHOULI**	*Very intense, woody, sweet, balsamic*	Base: strong Middle: strong Top: mild	✳	Oil is extracted from the dried leaves by steam distillation. Cultivated in Southeast Asia, India, and the West Indies.
Pinus sylvestris **SCOT'S PINE**	*Medicinal, turpentine-like, balsamic*	Base: weak Middle: weak Top: strong	✳	Oil is extracted from the needles and cones by steam distillation. Cultivated in Finland, Norway, and Siberia.
Vetiveria zizanoides **VETIVER**	*Rich, warm, smoky, woody, popular with men*	Base: strong Middle: strong Top: mild	✳ ✳	Oil is extracted from the roots by steam distillation. Cultivated in India, Haiti, the island of Réunion, and Comoro Islands.
Canaga odorata **YLANG YLANG**	*Heady, floral, tenacious, exotic*	Base: mild Middle: strong Top: strong	✳ ✳	Oil is extracted from the flowers by steam distillation. Cultivated in the Comoro Islands, Madagascar, and the island of Réunion.

Main Constituents	Therapeutic Properties	Common Uses	Cautions (see page 16)
Vanillin, benzoic acid	*Warming and soothing; expectorant; promotes skin healing*	• In inhalations for respiratory problems • Ingredient in hand creams to help heal dry, cracked skin	• May irritate skin because of solvent extraction • Avoid on babies
Pinene, piperine, limonene, sabinene	*Stimulates blood flow to the skin, therefore warming*	• In massage blends to warm before sports and to prevent stiffness afterward • In abdominal massage blends to combat digestive problems and constipation	• May irritate skin • Use low or very low dilutions (1% or less)
Cedrene, atlantone, cedrol, cadinene	*Stimulating; antiseptic; a general tonic*	• Ingredient in preparations for oily skin • In compresses to relieve rashes and itching • In scalp massage blends to combat dandruff and hair loss	• May irritate and sensitize skin • Use low or very low dilutions (1% or less) • Avoid in pregnancy
Gingerin, gingerol, zingerone, zingiberene, linalool, camphene	*Warming and stimulating*	• In chest rubs for respiratory problems • In massage blends for muscular aches • In compresses for arthritic or inflamed joints and bruises	• May sensitize skin • Use low dilutions (1%) • Avoid on face and neck, and on babies and children
Limonene, pinene, citral, bergaptene, camphene	*Cleansing and refreshing; antiseptic and astringent; a tonic*	• Ingredient in toners for greasy or acne-prone skin • In vaporizers to refresh	• Avoid steam inhalations, sun and sunlamps for 6 hours • Use low dilutions (1%)
Citral, limonene, geraniol, methyl anthranilate	*Calming, refreshing, and uplifting; a tonic*	• In massage blends for nervous tension • In compresses for rheumatic aches • In massage blends to help relieve fluid retention and cellulite	• Avoid sun and sunlamps for 6 hours
Patchoulol, patchoulene	*Anti-inflammatory and bactericidal; a tonic; said to be an aphrodisiac*	• In massage blends for skin conditions, such as acne and eczema, and for aging skin, dandruff, and oily hair	• May cause headaches
Monoterpenes, bornyl acetate, cadinene, pinene, sylvestrene	*Invigorating; antiseptic; stimulates blood flow to the skin, therefore warming*	• In inhalations for coughs, colds, phlegm, and nasal congestion • In massage blends for stiffness and aches • In vaporizers to fight airborne microbes	• May irritate skin • Use low or very low dilutions (1% or less)
Vetiverol, vitivone, terpenes	*Strong sedative; calming; antiseptic*	• In massage blends for insomnia • In compresses for acne • Ingredient in aftershave lotions	• Strong sedative; avoid if driving • Often adulterated
Linalool, geraniol, pinene, benzyl acetate	*Sedative; induces feeling of well-being*	• In massage blends for stress • Ingredient in perfumes and hair- and skin-care preparations • Ingredient in pampering bath products	• May cause headaches and nausea • Use low dilutions (1%)

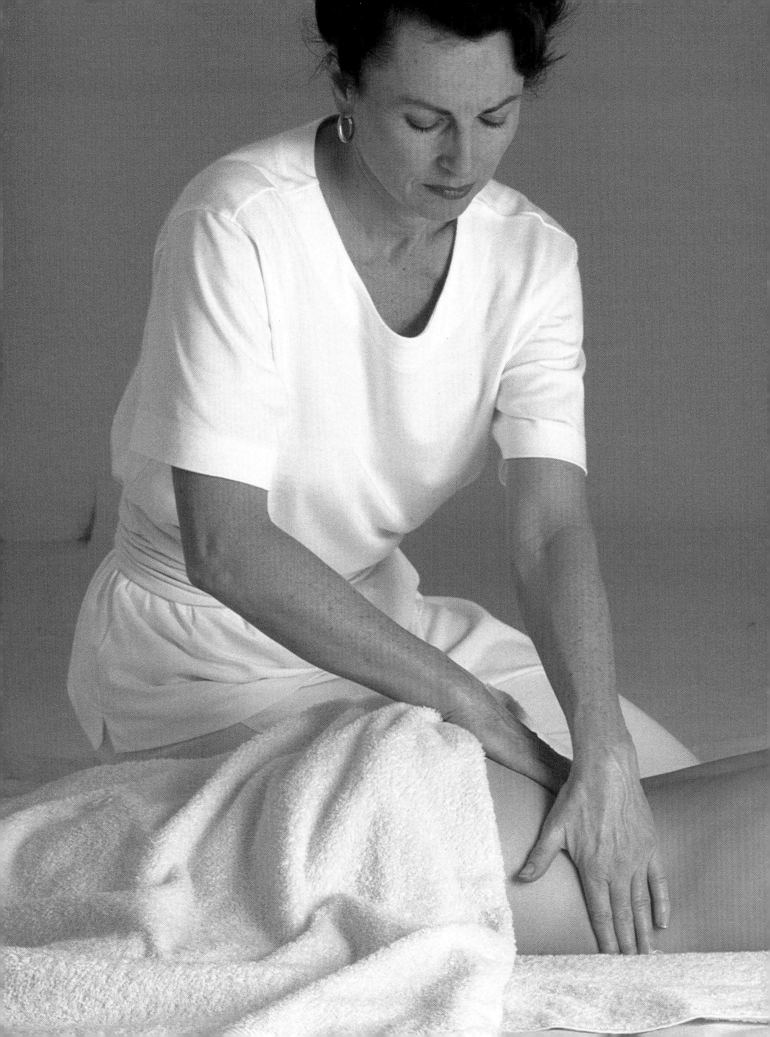

MASSAGE TECHNIQUES

My personal motto is "Life takes it out of you, but massage puts it back." The basis of massage is touch — and, to thrive, we all need the warmth and security touch engenders. On the following pages I demonstrate all the basic massage strokes and show how to combine them in a relaxing full body massage.

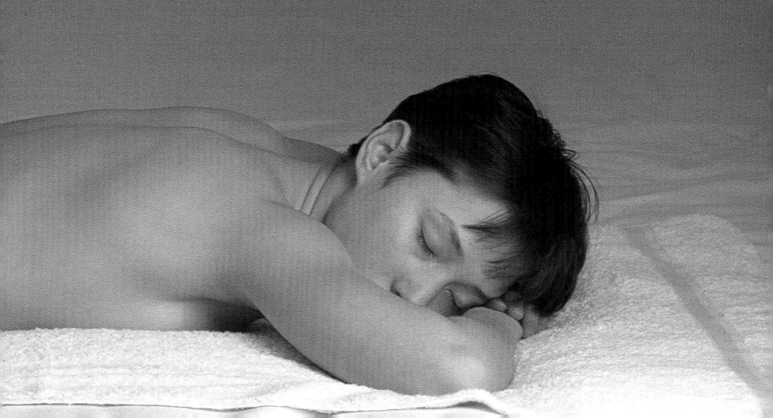

PREPARING TO MASSAGE

A massage with scented oils should be as relaxing to give as it is to receive, with one movement flowing into the next, leaving you and your partner calm. As with any new skill, massage takes practice. Try to persuade a friend to learn at the same time, so that you can help one another develop your massage technique. During a massage, it is essential that both you and your partner feel at ease, so start by making your environment as comfortable as possible.

ENVIRONMENT

Choose a peaceful, quiet, warm room with subdued lighting. I like to work on the floor, padded with a futon or a couple of thick blankets, as it provides plenty of space to spread out. To prevent sore knees, kneel on a cushion and change your position often. You can also work on a sturdy, well-padded kitchen table, or you may wish to invest in a massage couch, especially if you tend to get a tired back or if kneeling for prolonged periods causes you discomfort. Most traditional beds are too soft for massage and absorb all your strength. Cover the table or floor with towels. I place a small electric blanket or hot water bottle under the towels, and the gentle heat keeps my clients warm.

YOUR COMFORT

Wear loose, comfortable clothing, remove jewelry, and make sure your nails are short. To give a good massage, you need to be fully absorbed in what you are doing. Concentrate on your friend, breathe deeply, and enjoy the rhythm of the movements – your sense of tranquillity will be transmitted to your friend. Keep your back as straight as possible during the massage, and use your body weight, instead of force, to vary the depth of the movements. Learn to be sensitive and to "listen" with your hands. To increase flexibility, squeeze a rubber ball in each hand, flexing and extending your fingers, for a minute a day.

PAMPERING YOUR FRIEND

Your friend's general health and what he or she hopes to gain from the massage will govern your choice of essential oils. For instance, is stress a problem? Does your friend need to feel wide awake at the end of the treatment, or is there time to sleep afterward? Discuss contraindications (see Warnings below), and then select an appropriate blend of essential oils from pages 17–39, ensuring that he or she likes the aroma. Once your friend has undressed, cover the body with plenty of large towels to keep in warmth and enhance the feeling of comfort. It is surprising how cold one can become just lying still, and this makes it impossible to relax.

WARNINGS

Before starting to massage, ask whether your friend is pregnant or epileptic. If so, see the advice on page 16.

Never massage someone with any of the following conditions without a doctor's consent:

• Inflammatory conditions, such as varicose veins, thrombosis, or phlebitis

• Acute back pain, especially if the pain shoots down the arms or legs when you touch the back

• Skin infection, bruising, or acute inflammation

• Infection, contagious disease, or high fever

• Any other serious medical condition.

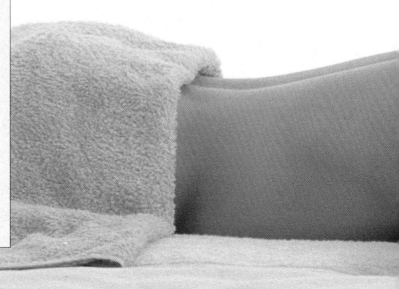

USING MASSAGE OIL

OIL HELPS THE HANDS glide smoothly over the body. For a full body massage, you will need about 4 tsp (20 ml) of carrier oil, to which you can add a few drops of essential oil (see page 15). The amount you use will depend on the size of your friend and the dryness of the skin. Shake the bottle, then warm a little oil between your hands. Keep the open bottle within reach in case you need more during the massage. If you do, keep one hand on the body while picking up the bottle.

APPLYING THE OIL

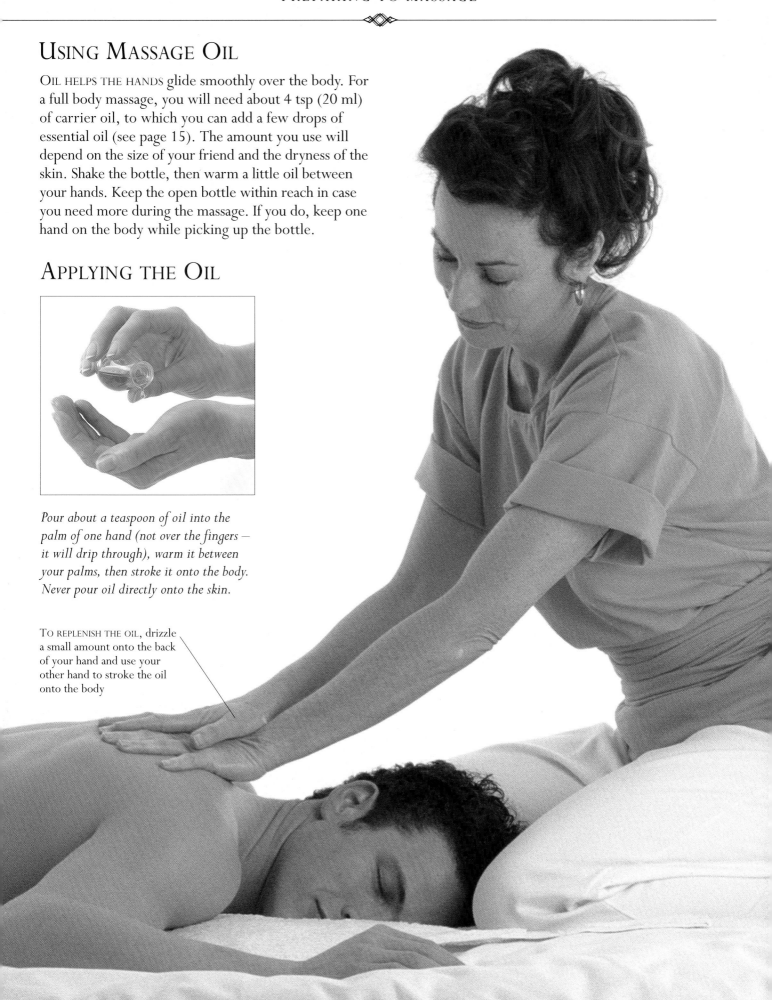

Pour about a teaspoon of oil into the palm of one hand (not over the fingers — it will drip through), warm it between your palms, then stroke it onto the body. Never pour oil directly onto the skin.

TO REPLENISH THE OIL, drizzle a small amount onto the back of your hand and use your other hand to stroke the oil onto the body

BASIC MASSAGE STROKES

Once you have mastered the basic strokes, you can use them all over the body and tailor each massage to suit the individual needs of your partner. Before you start practicing a new movement, read through the instructions and concentrate on learning just a few strokes at a time. To avoid awkward twisting, face the area you are massaging, and keep your back as straight as possible. Direct your strokes toward the heart, using your body weight to add depth.

FAN STROKING

Stroking movements are among the easiest and most calming to give and receive in massage, and you will probably return to them often to calm your friend and relax yourself. Use fan stroking to apply oil and to link different areas of the body, and when your hands are tired or you are deciding which movement to use next. Work smoothly and rhythmically. You can vary the length of the stroke, but keep the rhythm fluid.

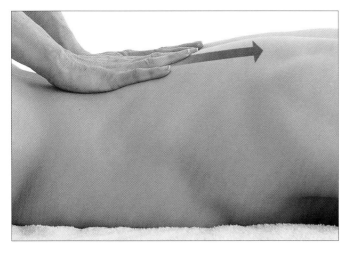

1 Place your hands side by side on the body, palms down, and then smoothly and gently glide upward, leading with your fingers. Keeping a straight back, lean forward on your hands, using the weight of your body to apply a steady, even pressure through the palms and heels of the hands.

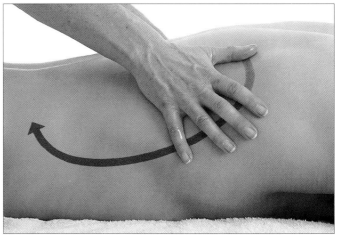

2 Fan your hands out to both sides of the body, reducing the pressure, and slide them down the sides, molding them to the contours of the body. Pull your hands up toward each other, and swivel them around to begin the upward movement again. Repeat several times, covering the whole area.

ALTERNATE FAN STROKING

Follow the sequence above, using each hand alternately to stroke the body. This slight variation creates pleasant diagonal stretches. Starting with the right hand, stroke firmly upward and out. Then repeat the movement with the left hand so that it strokes up as the right hand glides down. Repeat several times to cover the whole area.

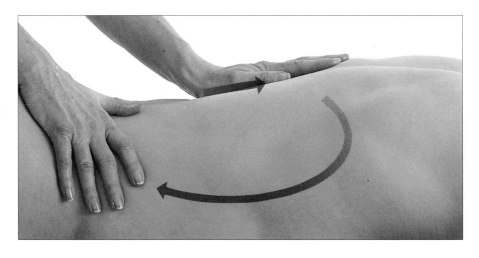

CIRCULAR STROKING

In this variation of fan stroking, both hands work on the same side, one hand completing a full circle while the other makes a half circle, building up a smooth and steady rhythm. Circular stroking is particularly effective on large areas, such as the back, shoulders, and abdomen. Like fan stroking, it is good for linking different areas in a full body massage. It produces a continuous flowing effect.

1 Place both hands, fingers pointing away from you, on one side of the body about 6 inches (15 cm) apart.

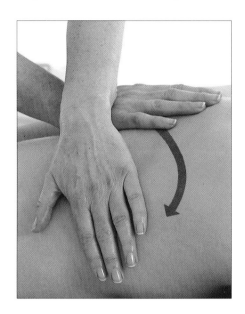

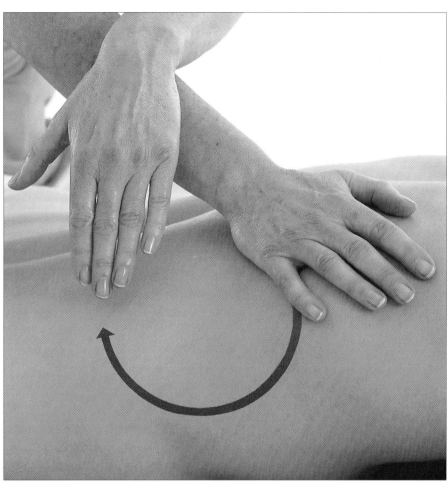

2 △ Begin to circle your hands in a clockwise direction, starting with the left hand, and following with the right.

3 △ As your left hand meets your right arm, lift your hand over, rejoining the body on the other side to finish the circle.

Repeat several times, stroking firmly on the upward and outward movement, and gliding gently to complete the circle.

THUMB STROKING

This firm movement is particularly useful on small, tense areas, such as the top of the shoulders and the neck. Alter the pressure to suit your friend's needs. If the muscles are very tight, begin gently, then stroke more firmly. To vary the effect, circle your thumbs, following steps 1–3 above for circular stroking.

With your hands resting on the body, stroke firmly upward and out to the side with your left thumb. Follow with the right thumb, stroking a little higher. Make the stroke smooth and repetitive, building up a steady rhythm.

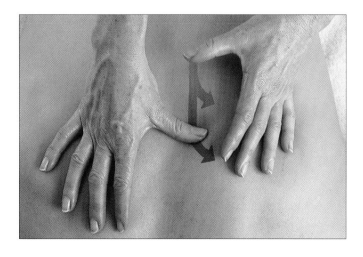

BASIC KNEADING

In a relaxing massage, kneading should be flat and smooth to produce an amazingly soothing effect. The movement is like kneading dough and is useful on the shoulders, back, and fleshy areas such as the hips. In Sarawak, Malaysia, on the island of Borneo, I learned to appreciate how soporific kneading can be when performed rhythmically. Normala, a Malaysian physiotherapist, taught me the value of counting "and one, and two, and three, and four, and five" over and over as I slowly kneaded. The repetition is very calming.

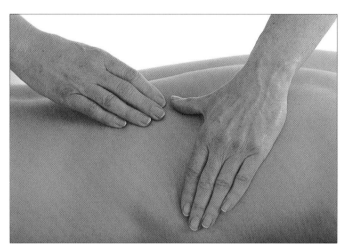

1 Place your hands flat on the body with your elbows apart, and fingers pointing away from you. With your right hand, gently grasp some flesh and release it into your left hand.

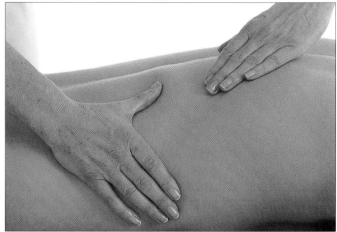

2 Let your left hand take the flesh and then release it into your right hand. Repeat several times, counting to keep your strokes rhythmic, like waves washing over the muscles.

CIRCULAR PRESSURES

Deep, penetrating circles are useful for exploring the state of the muscles and for combating tension. Apply the pressure gradually, beginning to circle more deeply and firmly, then slowly release and move on to the next area. For tight, knotted muscles, place one thumb on top of the other, and lean into the body.

STATIC PRESSURES

Stationary pressures are extremely useful for releasing tension in the neck and shoulders, sides of the spine, buttocks, and soles of the feet. Ease into the pressure gradually and steadily, hold, and then slowly release – never poke sharply. Treat the body with care, making sure that your fingernails do not gouge the skin.

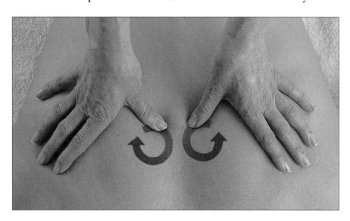

Using only a small amount of oil – too much will cause your thumbs to slide – place the pads of your thumbs on the skin and gradually lean into them. Press for a few seconds, then make small, penetrating, circular movements against the underlying muscle. Glide to the next area, and repeat the movement.

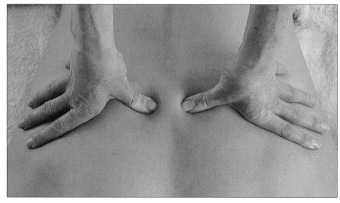

For this movement no oil is necessary. Place the pads of your thumbs on the skin and gradually lean into them. Hold for 5–9 seconds, then release slowly and glide to the next point of tension. Imagine how it feels to receive the massage – this helps your hands respond to the area you are working on.

KNUCKLING

For a heavenly sensation, rotate your knuckles on the shoulders, chest, palms of the hands, soles of the feet, and hips. You can work deeply without hurting.

Curl your hands into loose fists and, with the middle section of your fingers against the skin, ripple your fingers around in small, circular movements. Vary the pressure by leaning into the movement with more or less body weight. Work firmly and evenly to cover the entire tense area.

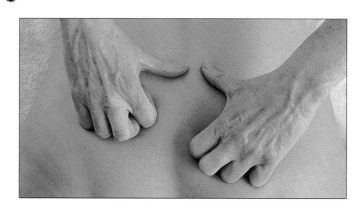

CAT STROKING

This is one of the nicest strokes with which to finish massaging an area. If done slowly and rhythmically it can soon send the recipient to sleep. Use a soft, gentle touch, and keep your movements smooth.

Place your left hand at the top of the area you are massaging and stroke slowly and lightly down the body, as if stroking a cat. Lift your hand off at the bottom of the area and return it to the start while the right hand begins the downward stroke. Repeat, making the return movement as smooth as the stroking.

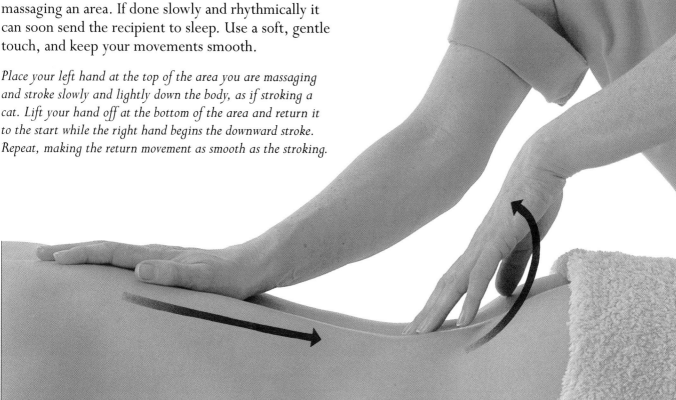

HOLDING

Many people love just being held – especially on the head, forehead, and abdomen. Simple holds are relaxing, comforting, and as calming for the person giving the massage as for the recipient.

Place one hand over the other, and gently hold. Concentrate on your partner's breathing and relax, releasing very slowly after one or two minutes. Never hurry this movement at the end of a massage: its effect will remain long after the massage finishes. If time is short, omit an earlier stroke rather than rushing this hold.

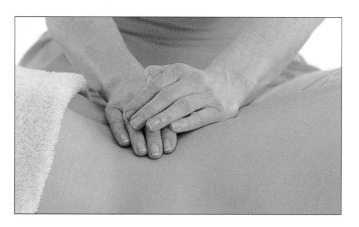

A FULL BODY MASSAGE

Massaging the whole body with aromatic oils has the power to release muscular tension, increase energy, and create a feeling of well-being. This massage starts on the back, moves down to the feet, and then continues on the front from head to toes. It takes about an hour and a half. Before you begin, discuss your friend's health to ensure that massage is safe (see page 42). Ask her to remove makeup, jewelry, and contact lenses. Remind her that she is in charge and must say if she feels uncomfortable.

THE BACK

EVERYBODY LOVES A BACK MASSAGE and, since most of the basic movements are used here, it is an ideal place to start. I begin by slowly stroking down the back to enhance relaxation. Work smoothly and rhythmically to create a hypnotic effect. If your hands get tired as you massage or you aren't sure what to do next, just stroke.

STARTING THE MASSAGE

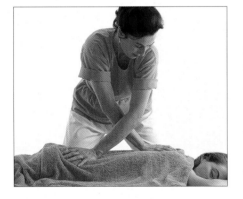

1 Kneel by your friend's left side. Place your left hand over the towel at the top of the back, and your right hand over the small of the back. Hold, breathing slowly to relax yourself and your friend.

2 ◁ Place your right hand on the left shoulder blade, and your left hand on the right hip. Lean forward to gently stretch the back. Repeat on the other side.

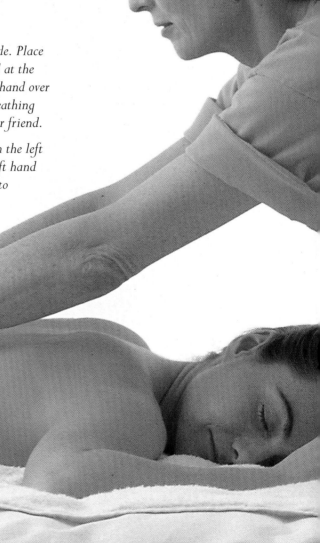

WHOLE BACK STROKING

 Choose an appropriate blend of essential oils (see pages 17–39) and mix them in a carrier oil.

1 ▽ *Fold the towel down. Sitting behind your friend's head, apply about a teaspoon of oil, as shown on page 43. Only apply more oil if your hands drag the skin. Place one hand on either side of the spine at the top of the back, and stroke down the back extremely slowly as far as you can reach.*

2 *At the base of the spine, fan your hands out over the hips and mold them around the sides of the back as you glide up to the shoulders and around the tops of the arms.*

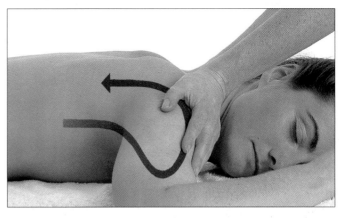

3 *Press down slightly as your hands swivel around the shoulders, before stroking smoothly down the back again, on either side of the spine. Repeat steps 1–3 several times to give your friend a wonderful, all-engulfing sensation.*

KEEP YOUR BACK STRAIGHT – the more comfortable and relaxed you are, the better your massage will be

KNEELING BEHIND your friend's head allows you to direct your strokes downward

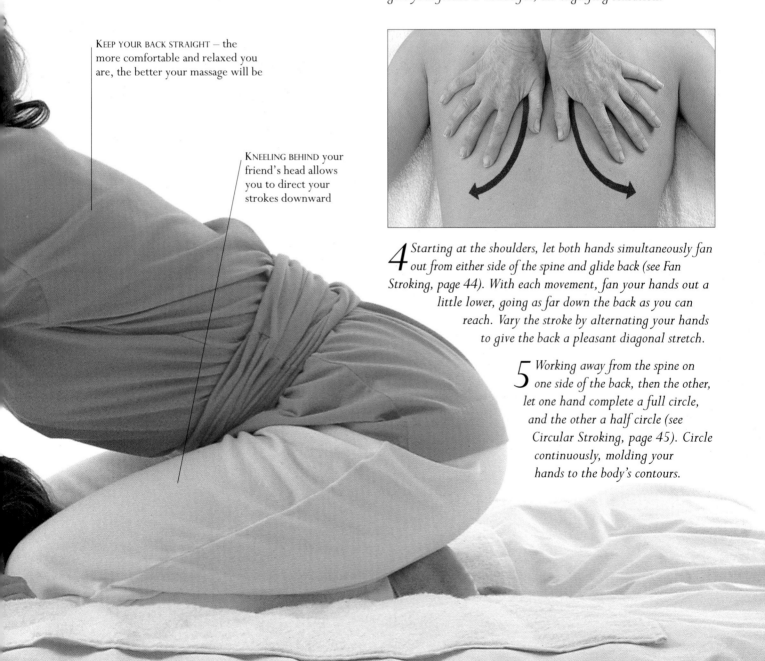

4 *Starting at the shoulders, let both hands simultaneously fan out from either side of the spine and glide back (see Fan Stroking, page 44). With each movement, fan your hands out a little lower, going as far down the back as you can reach. Vary the stroke by alternating your hands to give the back a pleasant diagonal stretch.*

5 *Working away from the spine on one side of the back, then the other, let one hand complete a full circle, and the other a half circle (see Circular Stroking, page 45). Circle continuously, molding your hands to the body's contours.*

FIGURE EIGHTS

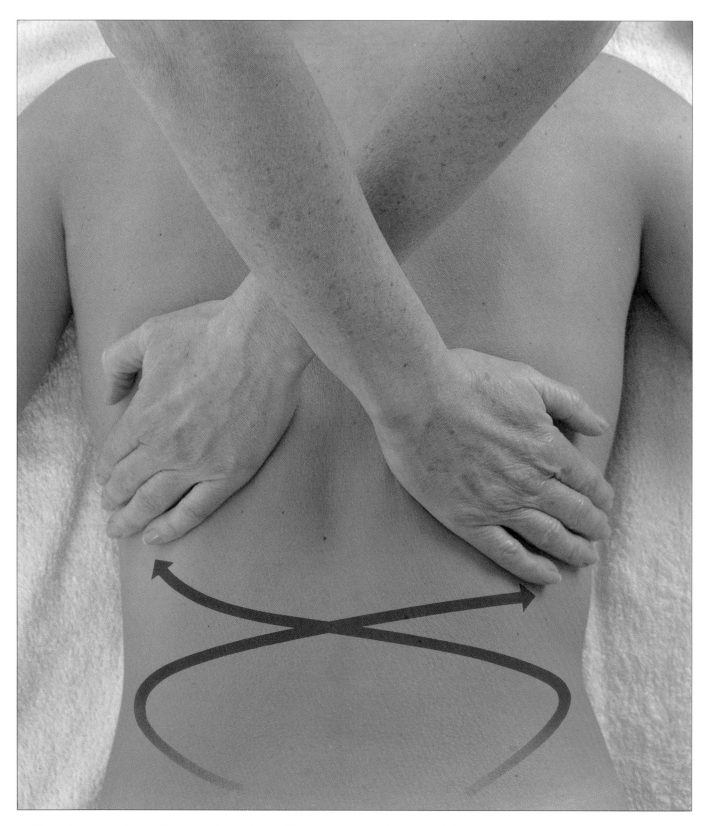

1 This relaxing stroke is a favorite with my clients. With one hand on each side of the spine at shoulder level, stroke firmly down to the small of the back. Fan out over the hips.

2 △ Now glide back up, crisscrossing the body to form a series of figure eights. Pull up at the sides and release as you cross the spine — never press on the spine. Repeat three times.

WORKING MORE DEEPLY

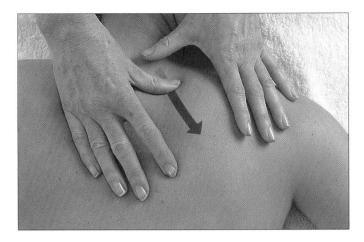

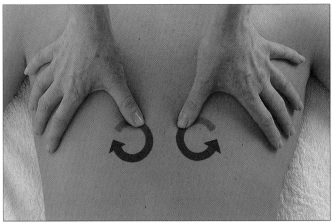

1 *Stroking with one thumb following the other, work down the right side of the neck and out to the top of the shoulder, keeping the movement firm to release taut muscles and ease away tension. Repeat on the left side.*

2 *Make large, flat circles with your thumbs on either side of the spine, from the shoulders down to the small of the back. Alter the depth and size of the circles: smaller, deeper circles are more penetrating and effective on tense areas.*

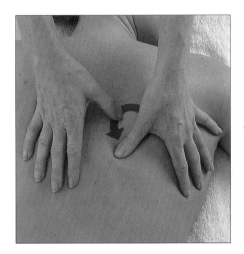

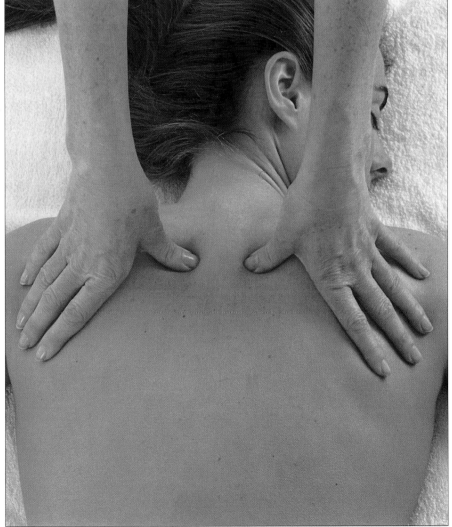

3 △ *Now place both thumbs on the right side of the spine by the shoulder. Make a full circle with one thumb and a half circle with the other, stroking away from the spine and working as far down the back as you can reach. This motion is similar to circular stroking (see page 45). Repeat on the left side.*

4 ▷ *Use static pressures (see page 46) on either side of the spine, from the base of the neck to the pelvis, on the tops of the shoulders, and on the scalp. Slowly lean on your thumbs, hold the pressure for 5—9 seconds, and release. Work slowly and carefully, using less weight on the neck, the base of the skull, and scalp.*

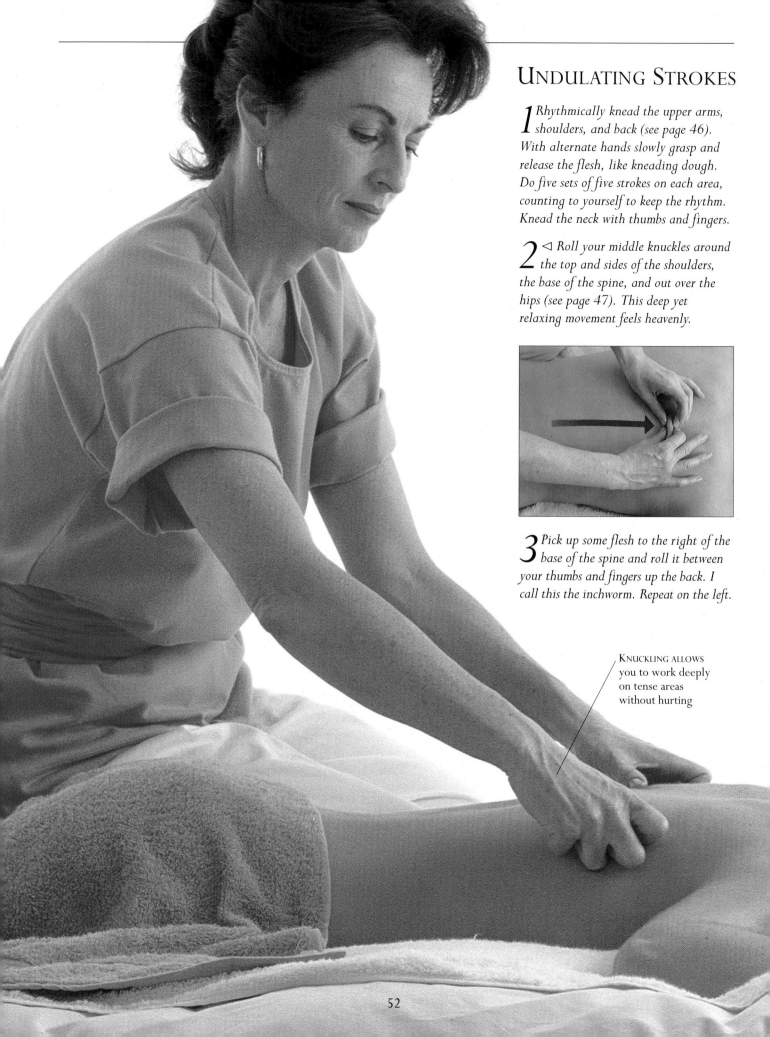

UNDULATING STROKES

1 Rhythmically knead the upper arms, shoulders, and back (see page 46). With alternate hands slowly grasp and release the flesh, like kneading dough. Do five sets of five strokes on each area, counting to yourself to keep the rhythm. Knead the neck with thumbs and fingers.

2 ◁ Roll your middle knuckles around the top and sides of the shoulders, the base of the spine, and out over the hips (see page 47). This deep yet relaxing movement feels heavenly.

3 Pick up some flesh to the right of the base of the spine and roll it between your thumbs and fingers up the back. I call this the inchworm. Repeat on the left.

KNUCKLING ALLOWS you to work deeply on tense areas without hurting

FINISHING TOUCHES

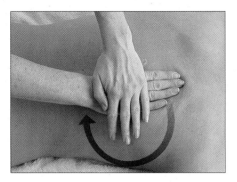

1 Place your left hand over your right to the right of the base of the spine, and make large, sweeping circles away from the spine up to the shoulder. Circle around the shoulder, relax the pressure and glide down to the lower left side. Then circle up the left side. Repeat several times. Then circle around the hips.

2 ▷ Keeping your left hand over your right, stiffen your arms and tense the muscles so that your hands vibrate gently as you stroke (without pressure) down from the top of the spine to its base. This small movement may take practice, but it is incredibly relaxing. Repeat twice.

3 Place your right hand on the neck, fingers pointing toward the head, and in a smooth, slow movement bring it down the spine and smoothly lift it off at the base as your left hand gently repeats the stroke. This hypnotic movement will make your partner feel like a stroked cat.

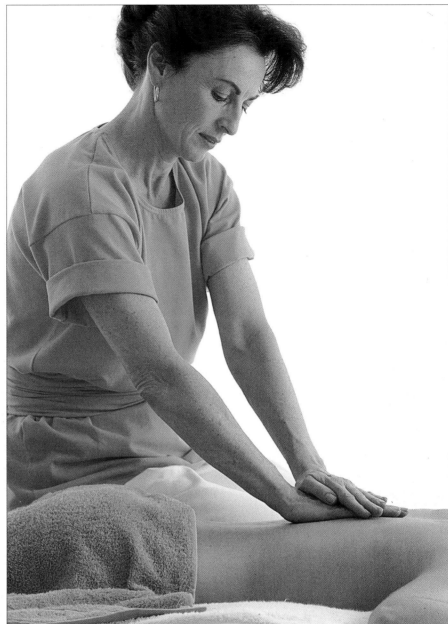

4 Rest your forearms horizontally across the middle of the back, with your wrists relaxed, and gradually stroke outward, your left arm going toward the head and your right arm toward the legs. Lean into this long stretch.

5 Cover your friend with a towel and finish the back massage with smooth rocking. With your left hand, hold the shoulder while your right hand gently rocks the small of the back to and fro. My clients frequently say this takes them back to their childhood and gives them a sense of security and peace.

THE BACK OF THE LEGS & FEET

FOLLOWING THE BACK MASSAGE, move down the body to begin work on the back of the legs and feet. Keep the rest of your friend's body covered with towels so that she stays warm while you massage first one leg, then the other. The movements described here help relieve tension and dispel fatigue while stimulating the circulation, and many of them can also be used on the front of the legs (see pages 64–5).

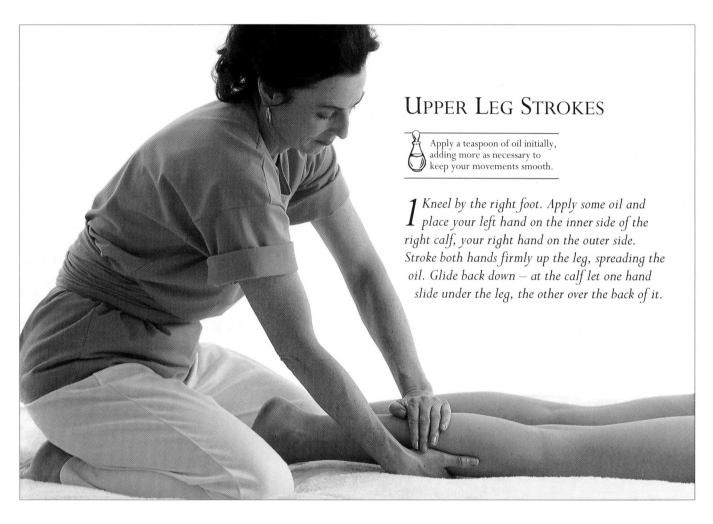

UPPER LEG STROKES

Apply a teaspoon of oil initially, adding more as necessary to keep your movements smooth.

1 *Kneel by the right foot. Apply some oil and place your left hand on the inner side of the right calf, your right hand on the outer side. Stroke both hands firmly up the leg, spreading the oil. Glide back down — at the calf let one hand slide under the leg, the other over the back of it.*

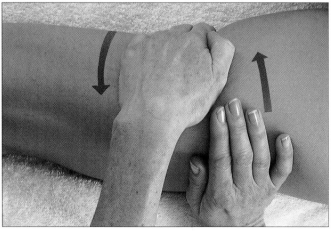

2 *Now kneel by your friend's right side, facing the thigh. Try to keep one hand in contact with the body while you move. Knead the thigh in rows (see page 46), keeping your hands open and relaxed. Count as you knead to maintain the rhythm.*

3 ◁ *Place your left hand on the inner thigh and your right hand on the outer thigh, and bring your hands together, pulling the flesh up toward the top of the leg. Release, then bring the flesh up from the other side, crisscrossing the leg.*

4 *Gently circle the thumbs of both hands over the back of the knee, without applying pressure. Gentle massage here is very soothing and helps stimulate the lymphatic system, which cleanses the body and returns water and proteins to the blood.*

LOWER LEG STROKES

1 Kneeling by your friend's feet, bend her right leg and rest the foot on your shoulder. Stroke from the ankle toward the knee with your palms, then knead the calf with alternating hands.

2 ▷ Stroke down the calf from ankle to knee with your right, then left forearm, and glide back. Repeat several times.

3 Lower the leg and circle your thumbs rhythmically around the ankle. Stroke the sole of the foot with your thumbs, and then circle around the heel.

4 Press the middle knuckles of both hands into the sole of the foot as if walking on it. Repeat three times. Then relax your friend by sandwiching the foot between your hands. Repeat the entire massage sequence on the left leg.

THE FACE

WHILE YOUR FRIEND TURNS over and settles under the towels, wash your hands and double-check that she has removed contact lenses. This simple face massage should only take about 15 minutes. Although it is easier to work with oil or cream, it is possible to do the massage without any lubricant if your partner doesn't want her hair to get oily. If you prefer, you can do this massage at the end of the full body massage.

Use just enough oil to allow your hands to move freely without slipping over the skin.

1 Sit behind your friend's head. If you use oil, apply it with your palms from the forehead to the neck. Then stroke out from the center of the brow to the temples. Repeat three times.

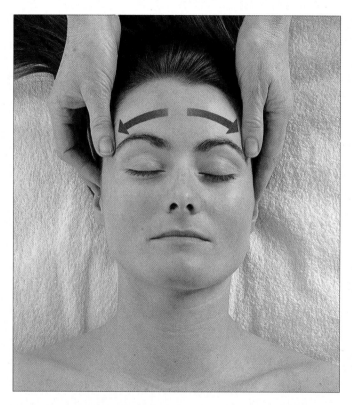

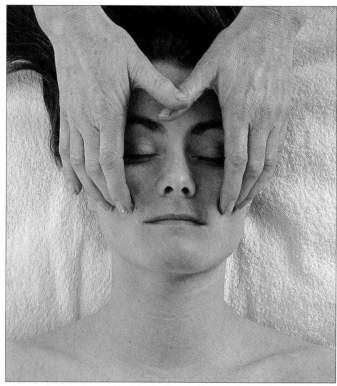

2 Using your thumbs, stroke from the center of the forehead out to the temples, working first at the hairline, then on the middle of the forehead, and finally on the eyebrows. Repeat the movement three times, gently stroking away tension.

3 With your thumbs, stroke from the forehead down the bridge of the nose, under the cheekbones, and up to the temples. Then apply gentle pressure with two fingers beside the nostrils, under the cheekbones, and at the temples. Repeat three times.

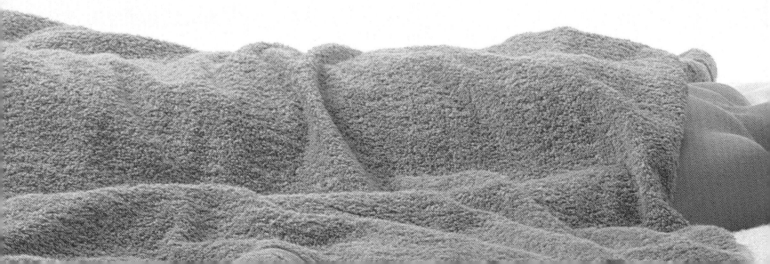

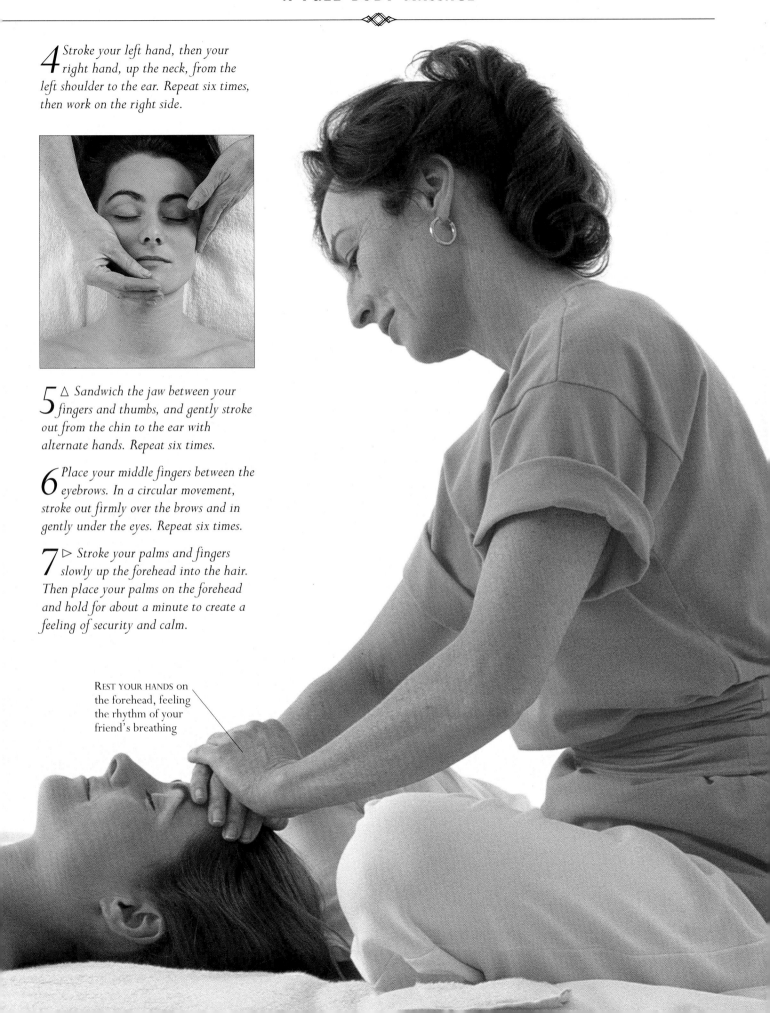

4 Stroke your left hand, then your right hand, up the neck, from the left shoulder to the ear. Repeat six times, then work on the right side.

5 △ Sandwich the jaw between your fingers and thumbs, and gently stroke out from the chin to the ear with alternate hands. Repeat six times.

6 Place your middle fingers between the eyebrows. In a circular movement, stroke out firmly over the brows and in gently under the eyes. Repeat six times.

7 ▷ Stroke your palms and fingers slowly up the forehead into the hair. Then place your palms on the forehead and hold for about a minute to create a feeling of security and calm.

REST YOUR HANDS on the forehead, feeling the rhythm of your friend's breathing

CHEST, SHOULDERS & NECK

ALMOST EVERYONE CARRIES TENSION in the shoulders and neck, so this is an extremely popular area to massage. By working on the chest, you relax the muscles and encourage deeper breathing. With your partner lying on her back, you can easily get your fingers behind the neck to massage either side of the spine and work on the base of the skull. As you use these gentle, hypnotic strokes, tension will melt away.

1 Kneel behind your friend's head and begin by massaging over the towel that covers her. Imagine that the heels of your hands are a cat's paws and "walk" over the chest. This rhythmic movement will help her relax.

Pour a small amount of oil into your palm, and remember to rub your hands together to warm it.

2 ▷ Fold down the towel. Apply some oil to your hands and place them on the collarbone; fan firmly out over the top of the chest and shoulders and gently push down, releasing as you complete the circle. Now circle out over the shoulders. Repeat six times.

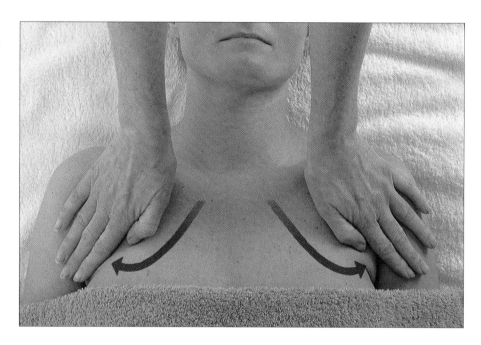

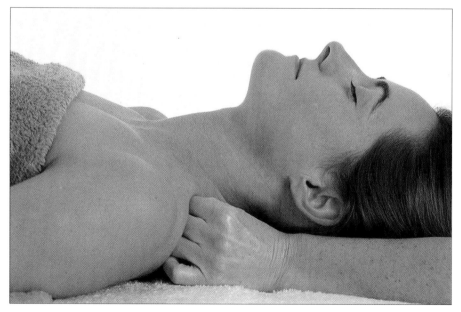

3 △ Rest your forearms on the floor and loosely rotate your fingers against the base of the neck, using your knuckles to loosen taut muscles. Anyone with tense shoulders will love this movement.

4 Stroke your hands up the back of the neck, and pull gently at the base of the skull to stretch the neck slightly. Release, and repeat the movement at least four times.

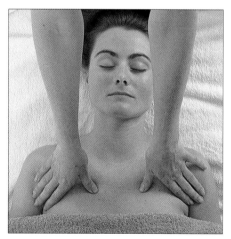

5 Stroke your thumbs out from the center of the chest, just below the collarbone, along the muscles between the ribs. Repeat the movement as far down as it is comfortable for your friend, avoiding the breasts. Ask your friend to tell you if she feels any discomfort.

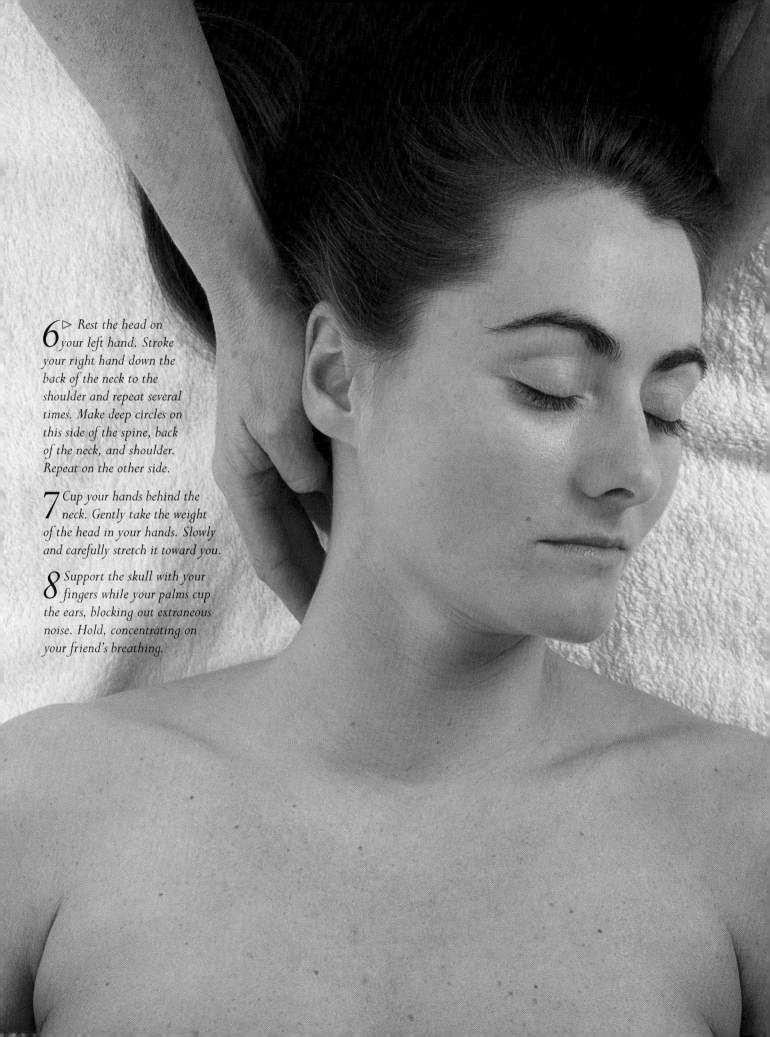

6 ▷ *Rest the head on your left hand. Stroke your right hand down the back of the neck to the shoulder and repeat several times. Make deep circles on this side of the spine, back of the neck, and shoulder. Repeat on the other side.*

7 *Cup your hands behind the neck. Gently take the weight of the head in your hands. Slowly and carefully stretch it toward you.*

8 *Support the skull with your fingers while your palms cup the ears, blocking out extraneous noise. Hold, concentrating on your friend's breathing.*

ARMS & HANDS

TENSION IN ONE AREA can often be released by stroking another part of the body, which is one of the reasons a complete body massage is so relaxing. If tense arms are causing the shoulders to ache, these calm, hypnotic movements will soothe and gently ease tension out of the muscles. Arm muscles are usually strong, so your movements here can be firm, while simply holding and stroking the hand can be calming and reassuring to your massage partner.

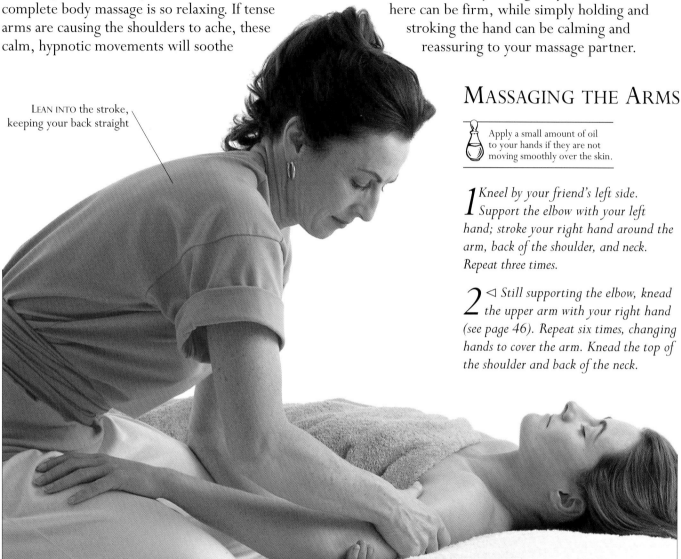

LEAN INTO the stroke, keeping your back straight

MASSAGING THE ARMS

Apply a small amount of oil to your hands if they are not moving smoothly over the skin.

1 Kneel by your friend's left side. Support the elbow with your left hand; stroke your right hand around the arm, back of the shoulder, and neck. Repeat three times.

2 ◁ Still supporting the elbow, knead the upper arm with your right hand (see page 46). Repeat six times, changing hands to cover the arm. Knead the top of the shoulder and back of the neck.

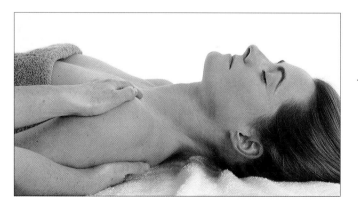

3 ◁ Place your left hand above the left shoulder, and slide your right hand underneath the body, hooking your fingers around the shoulder blade. Guide with your left hand while your right hand gently pulls toward you, stretching the muscles.

4 Stroke the entire arm, including the elbow. Support the wrist with your left hand, and with your right hand knead the lower arm slowly. Change hands to cover the whole area.

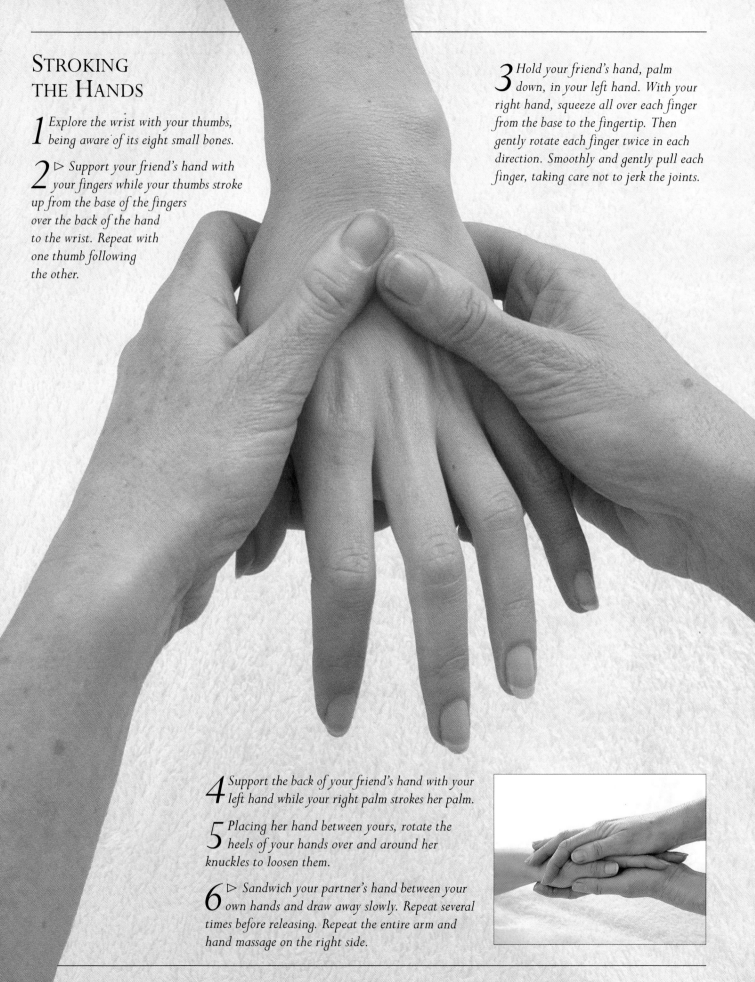

STROKING THE HANDS

1 Explore the wrist with your thumbs, being aware of its eight small bones.

2 ▷ Support your friend's hand with your fingers while your thumbs stroke up from the base of the fingers over the back of the hand to the wrist. Repeat with one thumb following the other.

3 Hold your friend's hand, palm down, in your left hand. With your right hand, squeeze all over each finger from the base to the fingertip. Then gently rotate each finger twice in each direction. Smoothly and gently pull each finger, taking care not to jerk the joints.

4 Support the back of your friend's hand with your left hand while your right palm strokes her palm.

5 Placing her hand between yours, rotate the heels of your hands over and around her knuckles to loosen them.

6 ▷ Sandwich your partner's hand between your own hands and draw away slowly. Repeat several times before releasing. Repeat the entire arm and hand massage on the right side.

THE ABDOMEN

GREAT SENSITIVITY IS REQUIRED when massaging the abdomen because many people are nervous about being touched here. Reassure your friend that your strokes will be gentle, and massage confidently in a clockwise direction, following the workings of the intestines. Smooth, repetitive massage with aromatic oils helps calm the nerves, combat constipation, and stimulate the digestive system while toning the skin.

1 Kneel by your friend's right side, facing the abdomen. Place your hands gently over the towels covering her, and slowly rock her abdomen back and forth to loosen the muscles and ease tension.

Pour about a teaspoon of oil into your palm, and rub your hands together to warm it.

2 ▷ Fold back the towels and apply some oil. Lightly rest your left hand on the rib cage or just below it, and with your right hand circle the navel in a clockwise direction. Circle smoothly and confidently, gradually getting firmer and building a steady rhythm. Then gently introduce the left hand to the stroke, so that both hands are circling the navel (see Circular Stroking, page 45). Stroke continuously, feeling the tension abate.

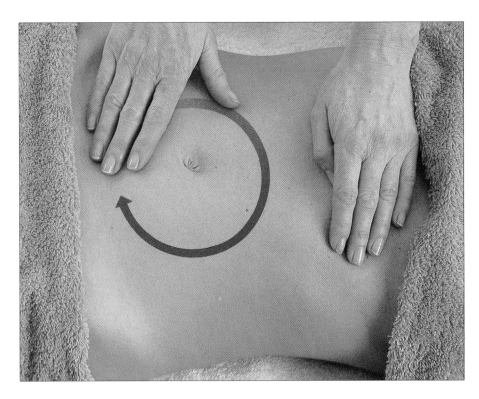

3 ◁ With your left hand on your right, make an undulating movement, gently pressing and releasing as you work in a triangle around the navel. Keep the movement fluid and rhythmic.

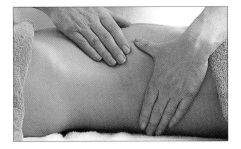

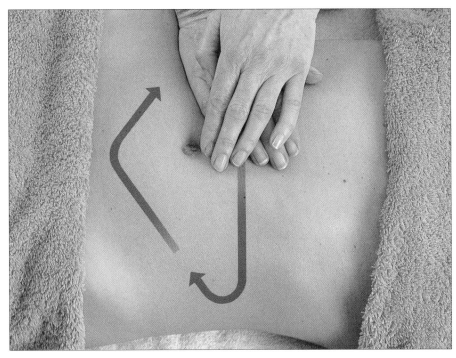

4 With flat, open hands, knead the far side of the abdomen, followed by the middle section, and then the near side (see page 46). Count while you knead to keep the rhythm constant.

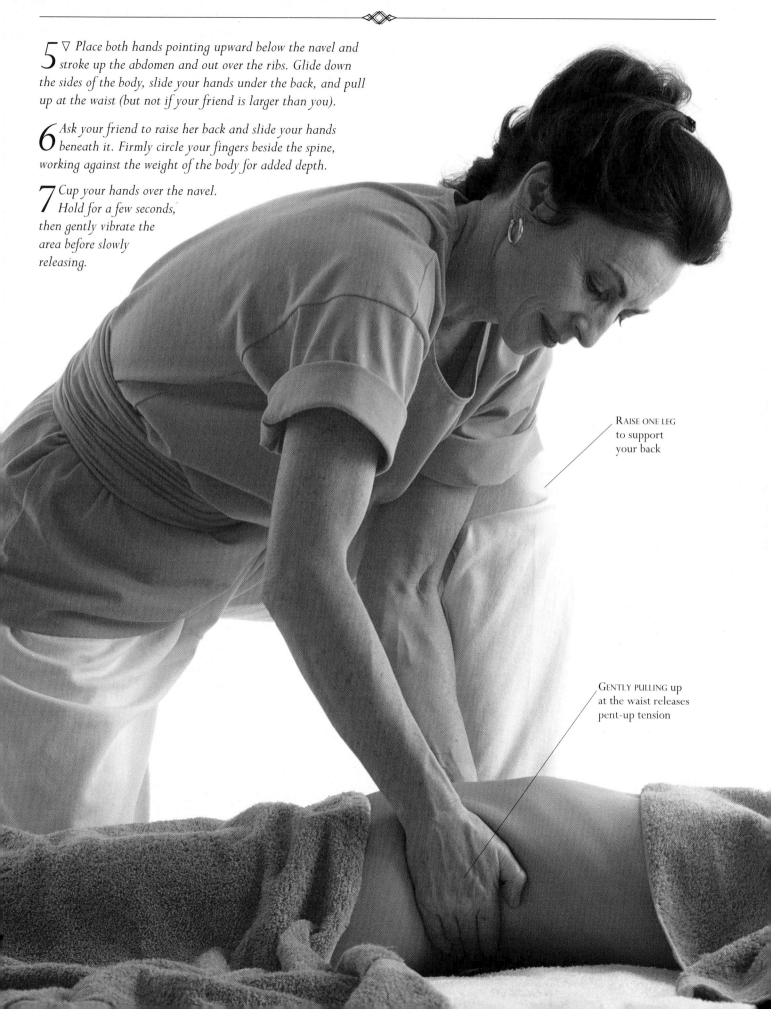

5 ▽ *Place both hands pointing upward below the navel and stroke up the abdomen and out over the ribs. Glide down the sides of the body, slide your hands under the back, and pull up at the waist (but not if your friend is larger than you).*

6 *Ask your friend to raise her back and slide your hands beneath it. Firmly circle your fingers beside the spine, working against the weight of the body for added depth.*

7 *Cup your hands over the navel. Hold for a few seconds, then gently vibrate the area before slowly releasing.*

RAISE ONE LEG to support your back

GENTLY PULLING up at the waist releases pent-up tension

THE FRONT OF THE LEGS

WHEN MASSAGING THE LEG, imagine that you are sculpting it into a perfect shape – this will help your strokes go in the right direction. Begin on the left leg, and then continue with the foot massage shown on pages 66–7 before returning to massage the right leg. These firm, repetitive movements stimulate the circulation, dispel fatigue, help relieve aches and pains, and can also be used before or after exercise.

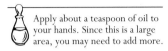 Apply about a teaspoon of oil to your hands. Since this is a large area, you may need to add more.

1 Kneel by the left foot and apply some oil to your hands. Place your left hand under the foot and your right hand on top, sandwiching it. Slide slowly and firmly up the leg and glide down. Repeat several times, building a rhythm.

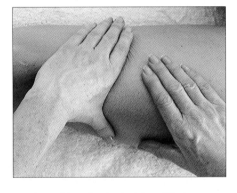

2 Kneel beside the left leg. With alternate hands, knead the thigh by methodically squeezing and releasing the flesh. Use firm strokes on the outer thigh and gentle strokes on the inner thigh.

LEAN INTO this simple but strong movement, using your body weight to add depth

3 Place one hand on either side of the thigh, fingers facing away from you, and firmly bring your hands toward each other. Release them on top of the leg and glide down the other side in a crisscross movement. Repeat six times.

4 Knuckle the thigh with both hands (see page 47), paying special attention to the outer thigh.

5 ▷ Keeping a V-shaped space between your index finger and thumb, stroke your left hand firmly up the thigh, then lift off to start again while your right hand begins the stroke. Repeat six times.

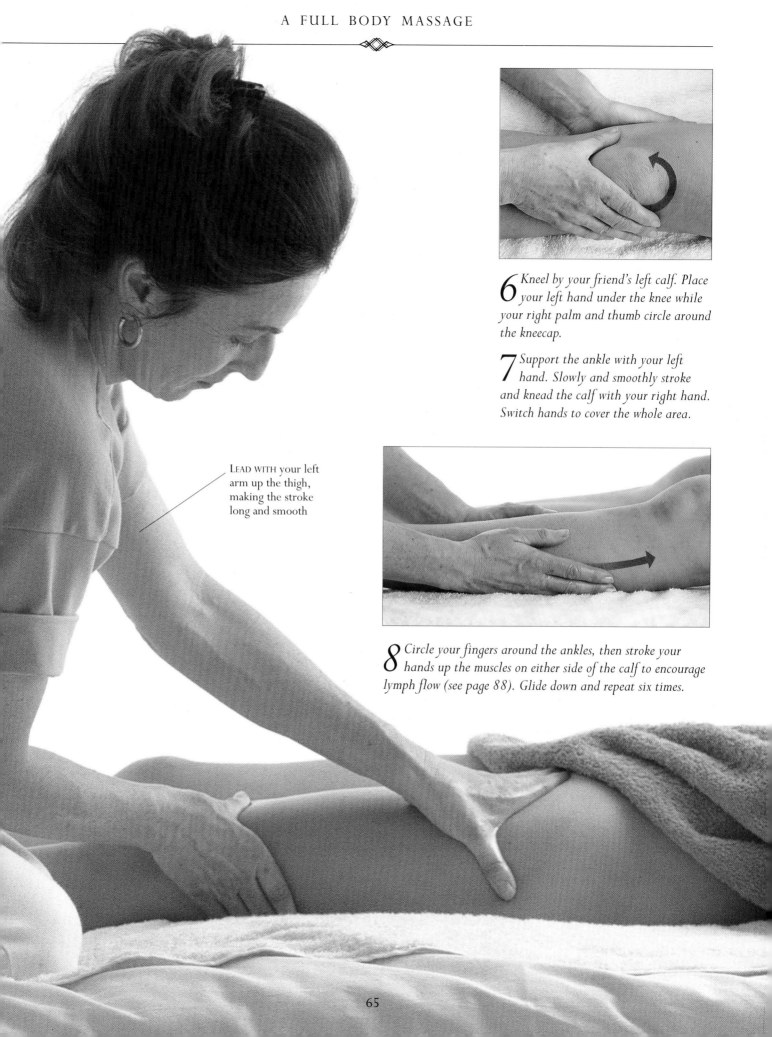

6 *Kneel by your friend's left calf. Place your left hand under the knee while your right palm and thumb circle around the kneecap.*

7 *Support the ankle with your left hand. Slowly and smoothly stroke and knead the calf with your right hand. Switch hands to cover the whole area.*

LEAD WITH your left arm up the thigh, making the stroke long and smooth

8 *Circle your fingers around the ankles, then stroke your hands up the muscles on either side of the calf to encourage lymph flow (see page 88). Glide down and repeat six times.*

THE FEET

MASSAGING THE FOOT with scented oils can be particularly relaxing and usually evokes sighs of delight. It relieves fatigue and revitalizes and relaxes the whole body. Because some people are ticklish on their feet and may be nervous at first, use confident, firm movements with just enough oil to allow your fingers to move smoothly.

Apply a small amount of oil – too much will cause your fingers to slip and slide.

1 Kneel in front of your friend's left foot. Apply a little oil to your hands. Supporting the foot with the fingers of both hands, stroke your thumbs from the base of the toes up to the ankle.

KEEP YOUR WRISTS LOOSE – the more relaxed you are, the better the massage will feel

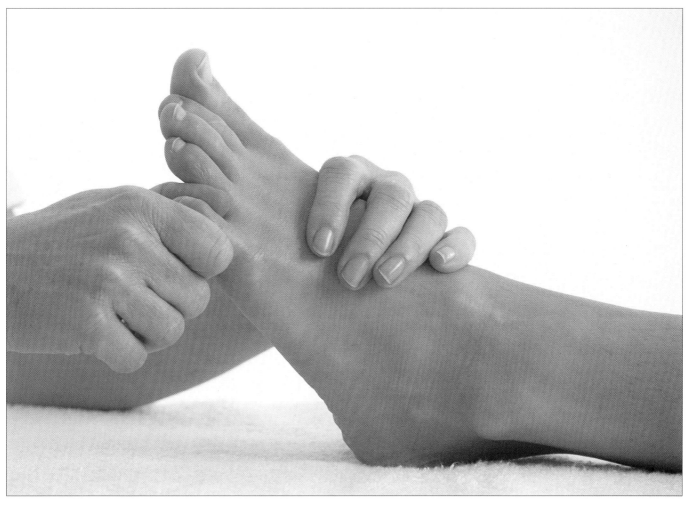

2 Support the foot with your left hand and use your right thumb and index finger to squeeze between the joints of each toe, feeling the underlying structure as you work. Massage *each toe individually, gently rolling, rubbing, and squeezing it all over, including the nail tip. Then carefully pull each toe toward you, slowly stretching it.*

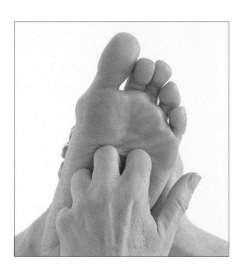

3 Rest your right hand on the top of the foot, and roll and press the knuckles of your left hand into the ball of the foot. Repeat three times.

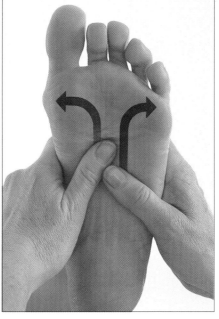

4 Still resting your right hand on top of the foot, stroke the heel of your left hand firmly down from the ball of the foot into the arch and then down to the heel. Repeat three times.

5 ◁ Supporting the foot with your fingers, stroke both thumbs firmly up the sole. At the ball of the foot, stroke out in a T-shape, glide back down toward the heel, and repeat six times.

6 Sandwich the foot between your hands and stroke several times up toward the body, then slowly draw your hands away. Repeat the sequence on the right leg and foot (return to page 64).

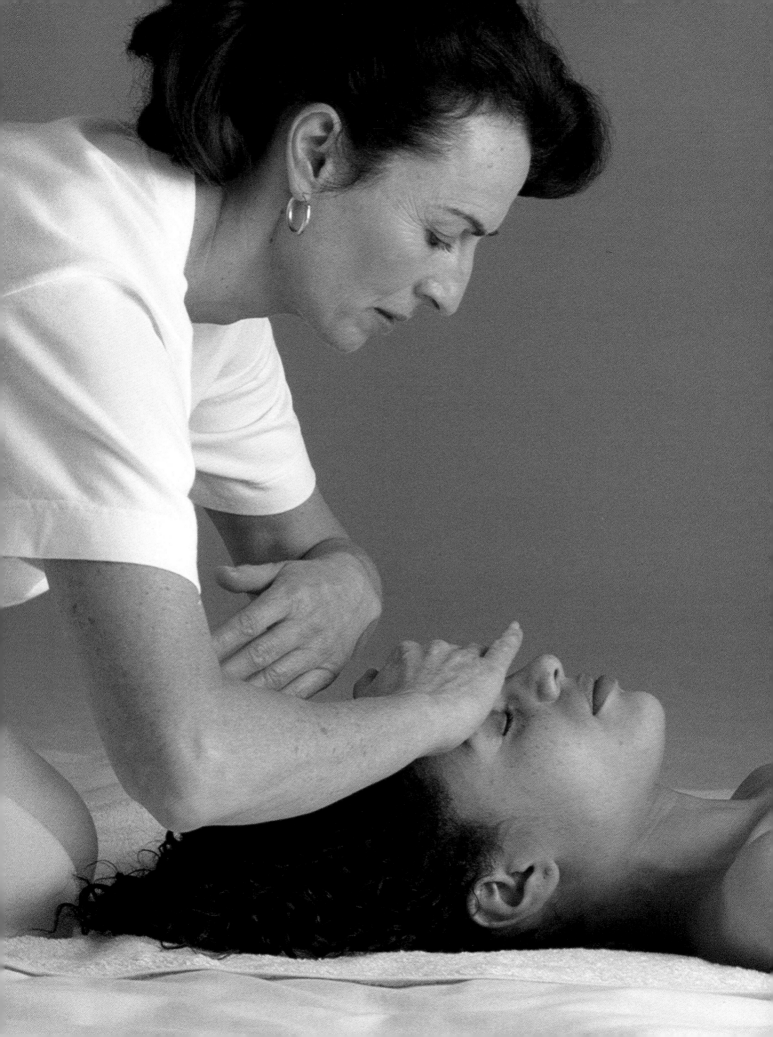

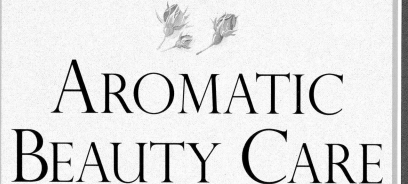

AROMATIC
BEAUTY CARE

Avicenna, the 10th-century philosopher and physician, claimed that diet, exercise, and sleep were the prerequisites for health. I believe that health and beauty are inextricably linked and that a few minutes' massage each day using the nourishing aromatherapy beauty preparations on the following pages makes skin care a pleasure.

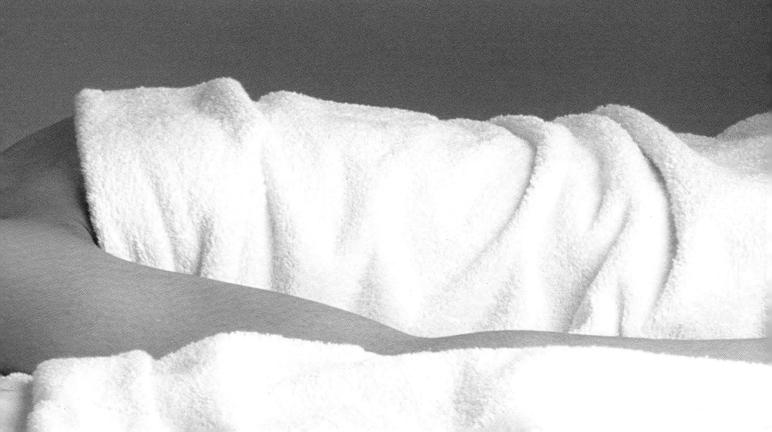

MAKING BEAUTY BASICS

My philosophy for skin care is simple: we do not need hundreds of exotic products, just a few that really work, including a cleanser, toner, moisturizer, mask, and massage oil or cream. I will never forget the excitement of making my first cosmetics – the process is as easy as basic cooking. It is also inexpensive and allows you to select essential oils with scents you enjoy and ingredients to suit your skin type. Like food, skin-care products should be prepared under hygienic conditions. If kept in a refrigerator, most should last at least a month.

THE FINISHED PRODUCTS

Cleansing grains   **Moisturizing cream**   **Pomade**   **Clay mask**   **Fruit mask**

INGREDIENTS & EQUIPMENT

For some recipes, special ingredients and equipment are required as well as essential oils (see pages 17–39), carrier oils (see page 14), and basic kitchen items.

SPECIAL INGREDIENTS

Fuller's earth: an earthy, hydrous aluminum silicate capable of absorbing grease
Green clay: the finest clay, for sensitive and dry skin
Kaolin: a fine white powder with a gentle astringent effect; use for normal or oily skin
Beeswax: a hard, waxy secretion from honeycomb
Lanolin: thick, sticky sebum from sheep's wool with a softening effect; use the anhydrous variety in the recipes

Cocoa butter: a solidified butterlike substance obtained from the roasted cocoa bean
Distilled water: water purified by distillation
Flower water: water infused with flowers

SPECIAL EQUIPMENT

Sterilized dark glass bottles: small (30 ml) and larger (100 ml) sizes for storing oils and toners
Sterilized jars: various sizes, (30–100 ml) for storing

creams, pomades, and cleansing grains
Heat-resistant bowls: small and medium sizes in which to mix ingredients
Funnels: to transfer oil or toner into bottles
Coffee filters: for filtering toners

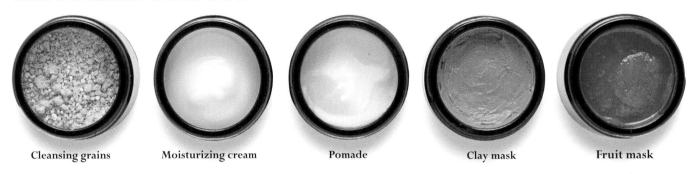

Lanolin

Beeswax

Funnels

Fuller's earth   Green clay   Kaolin   Cocoa butter   Glass jars and bottles   Filters

UNDERSTANDING YOUR SKIN

Skin, which is your protection against the elements, blocks out bacteria, and by perspiring eliminates waste and water. Under perfect conditions, the skin will be self-cleaning, self-lubricating, and self-renewing, but sun, wind, and harsh products disrupt these natural processes and can cause the following problems.

Dry skin is often fine and delicately textured and can feel as though it is pulled too tightly over the face. It has a tendency to develop broken capillaries and tiny lines which, if neglected, turn into wrinkles. To prevent premature aging and dehydration, generously use rich emollient creams and oils made with apricot kernel, avocado, sweet almond, and jojoba. Dry skin responds well to essential oils that encourage skin renewal, including benzoin, frankincense, jasmine, lavender, rose, and sandalwood.

Oily skin tends to look sallow and greasy and has a heavy, unrefined texture. The grease picks up dirt, clogging the pores, which can lead to blackheads and pimples. Keep oily skin meticulously clean and moisturize it only where it feels dry, usually avoiding the chin and nose area. Use sunflower-, soy-, or grapeseed-based creams and oils, containing geranium, bergamot, lavender, rosemary, or cypress for their antiseptic properties.

Combination skin is characterized by dry areas around the cheeks, neck, and eyes, and an oily T-shaped area on the forehead, nose, and chin. Balance the two types of skin by moisturizing the dry areas and always keeping the oily parts clean.

Sensitive skin can be of any type, and may become sensitive from rough handling or exposure to harsh products. Treat with simple sweet almond- or jojoba-based oils and creams containing soothing essential oils, such as chamomile.

Acne is caused by overactive sebaceous glands. Oil buildup blocks hair follicles, producing blackheads, while organisms living on the sebum break down into acids, causing swelling and pimples. Treat with diluted tea tree oil (see pages 108–9).

CLEANSING GRAINS

It is important to cleanse the skin gently to remove daily dirt and oil without stripping it of its natural oils. These washing grains have a gentle exfoliating effect and should be used once or twice a week instead of soap. Choose fine oatmeal for a mildly abrasive scrub, or medium oatmeal for a stronger, more abrasive scrub.

HONEY & OATMEAL WASHING GRAINS

Essential oils
12 drops (orange and geranium work well)
Base
1 cup oatmeal, fine or medium
$^1/_2$ cup ground almonds
10 ml sweet almond oil
1 tbsp clear honey

1 Put the oatmeal and almonds into a medium bowl. Set aside. In a small bowl, mix the oils and honey.

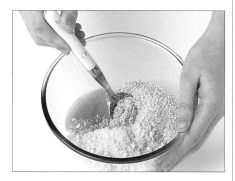

2 △ Add the oil mixture to the dry ingredients, stirring until well mixed. Transfer to a sterilized jar. To use, moisten a teaspoon of grains with a little rose water and rub gently over face. Rinse off.

AROMATIC OILS

This simple recipe makes a good cleanser, massage oil, and bath oil. Adjust the amounts to suit your needs: 5 ml is enough for a bath, 10 ml for the face, and 20 ml for a body massage; or make more and store for future use (see page 16).

BASIC OIL

Essential oils
6–10 drops (choose from 3–4 oils)
Carrier oil
20 ml to suit skin type (see above)

Pour the carrier oil through a funnel into a small, dark glass bottle. Add the essential oils, seal, and shake well.

OIL VARIATION

Relaxing oil to soothe jangled nerves: *add chamomile, clary sage, and marjoram essential oils to sweet almond carrier oil.*

TONERS

Skin toners and aftershave lotions, made by diluting essential oils in distilled water, leave the skin fresh, clean, and invigorated.

BASIC TONER

Essential oils
25 drops (choose from up to 4 oils)
Base
100 ml distilled water or flower water

1 Pour the water into a large, sterilized dark bottle. Add the essential oil and allow to stand for a month, shaking often.

2 Pour through a coffee filter-lined funnel into a large bottle. Shake.

BASIC AROMATIC VINEGAR

Essential oil
5–6 drops
Base
10 ml wine or cider vinegar, or vodka
80 ml distilled water

1 Pour the vinegar or vodka through a funnel into a small, sterilized dark bottle and add the essential oil. Allow to stand for a week, shaking the bottle daily.

2 Pour the toner through a coffee filter. Dilute with distilled water, and store in a large, sterilized dark bottle.

BASIC HONEY WATER

Essential oils
5 drops
Base
10 ml vodka
¼ tsp honey
80 ml distilled water or flower water

Mix the vodka, honey, and oils, and pour into a small, sterilized dark bottle. Allow to stand for ten days, shaking at times. Dilute with water. Store in a larger bottle.

VINEGAR VARIATION

Orange toner: in the basic toner recipe use 10 drops petitgrain, 10 orange, 5 neroli. Dilute with orange flower water.

CREAMS

Made of oils, waxes, and water, creams keep the skin pliable while providing protection against the elements. Select creams based on your skin type and preference. I believe that regular massage is the best way to apply cream, because it improves circulation and aids absorption. These recipes make about 100 ml of cream.

BASIC CREAM

Essential oil
4–6 drops
Base
7 gm beeswax
60 ml carrier oil
30 ml flower water
or distilled water

CREAM VARIATIONS

1 Light cream: in step 1, add 35 ml jojoba and use 10 gm beeswax and 45 ml carrier oil; in step 2, use 20 ml water.

2 Rich treatment cream: in step 1, add 15 gm lanolin, and use 45 ml carrier oil; in step 2, use 60 ml water.

3 Luxurious cream: in step 1, add 15 gm cocoa butter and use 45 ml carrier oil; in step 2, use 35 ml water.

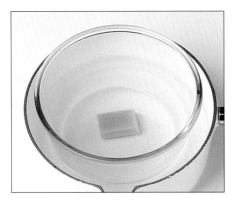

1 Put the beeswax and carrier oil into a heat-resistant bowl. Stir over a pan of boiling water until the mixture melts.

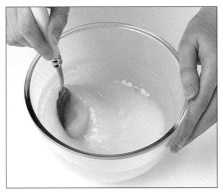

2 Remove the bowl from the pan, and slowly add the water to the mixture, stirring constantly.

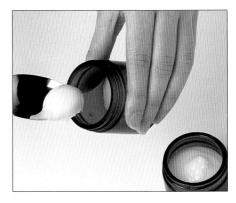

3 Keep stirring while the cream begins to cool, then add the essential oil. Stir until the mixture has thickened, then transfer it to sterilized jars.

POMADES

A pomade is a thick, rich mixture of oil and wax that has a wonderfully softening and smoothing effect on dry hands and feet. Choose carrier oils according to your skin type (see page 71). Because it contains no water, a pomade can be stored for more than a month in a refrigerator.

BASIC POMADE

Essential oil
20 drops
Base
15 gm beeswax
100 ml carrier oil
4 tbsp lanolin (optional, for dry skin)

1 Measure the beeswax, carrier oil, and lanolin into a heat-resistant bowl. Stir over a pan of boiling water until melted.

2 Remove the bowl from the pan. Keep stirring while the mixture begins to cool, then add the essential oil. When thickened, transfer to sterilized jars.

MASKS

Masks rejuvenate, soothe, and refine the skin. I recommend deep-cleansing clay masks for acne and other skin problems. They tighten as they dry, making skin glow. Non-drying masks can be made from yogurt, effective for treating acne and pimples, or from most fruit. AHAs (alpha hydroxy acids) in fruit have been hailed as antiwrinkling agents: by exfoliating the skin and boosting its ability to retain water, they smooth out lines. If you are allergic to a fruit, do a patch test first: place some on your wrist, and after 30 minutes rinse with cool water. If there is a reaction, avoid.

BASIC CLAY MASK

Essential oil
1 drop
Base
1 tsp fuller's earth, kaolin
or green clay
up to 5 ml flower water or
distilled water

1 Put the fuller's earth, kaolin, or green clay into a small bowl, then stir in flower or distilled water to make a paste.

2 Add the essential oil and mix well. Apply the mask to clean skin, avoiding the delicate area around the eyes, and wash off thoroughly after ten minutes.

MASK VARIATIONS

*1 **Nourishing fruit mask**: follow the basic fruit mask recipe, but in step 1 substitute avocado for fruit and add 1 tsp honey, 1 egg yolk, and 2 drops lemon juice.*

*2 **Soothing fruit mask** to counteract the damaging effects of the sun: follow the basic fruit mask recipe, using papaya in step 1 and 1–2 drops orange essential oil in step 2.*

*3 **Richer drying mask**: follow the basic clay mask recipe, adding 2 ml jojoba in step 1.*

BASIC FRUIT OR YOGURT MASK

Essential oil
1 drop
Base
1 tbsp ripe fruit or
1 tsp plain live yogurt

1 ▷ Mash the fruit and strain it into a small bowl. If using yogurt, simply place it in the bowl.

2 Add the essential oil and mix well. Apply the mask to clean skin, avoiding the delicate area around the eyes, and wash off after ten minutes.

STRAIN THE FRUIT into a bowl before adding the essential oil to the fruit mask

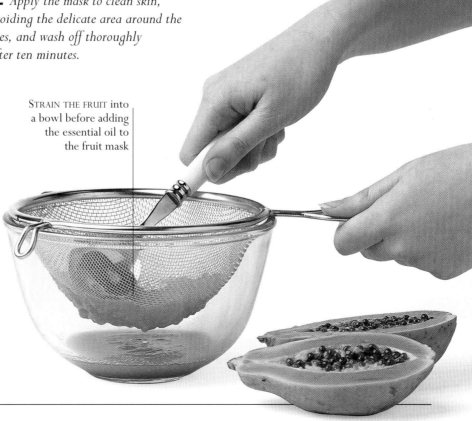

AROMATIC FACIAL

One of life's great luxuries, an aromatic facial with scented oil or cream improves skin tone while reducing tension and easing away worry lines. Men and women alike enjoy its delights. The massage movements stimulate the blood circulation and bring nourishment to the skin to encourage cell renewal and the elimination of waste. This truly pampering treatment leaves you feeling, and looking, years younger with glowing, healthy skin.

CLEANSING TREATMENT

Begin by applying a cleanser with smooth, gliding strokes to remove surface dirt. To relax the face and soften the skin, follow this with a hot, damp facecloth treatment. Soak the cloth in hot water containing an herbal tea bag (peppermint for oily skin or chamomile for dry or sensitive skin) or in hot water containing a drop of essential oil diluted in a teaspoon of carrier oil. This will open the pores for the massage.

SIMPLE CLEANSING OIL

Essential oils
5 drops lavender, 4 drops orange
Carrier oil
30 ml grapeseed, sunflower, or soy

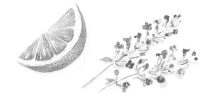

Follow method for basic oil, page 71.

LAVENDER CLEANSING CREAM

Essential oil
4 drops lavender
Base
7 gm beeswax, 60 ml sunflower oil
30 ml orange flower water

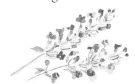

Follow method for basic cream, page 72.

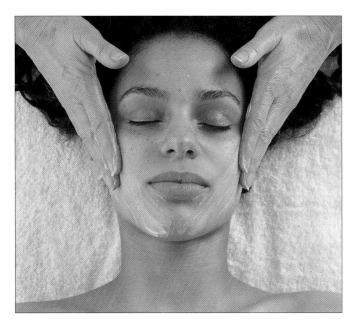

1 Make sure your friend removes contact lenses and jewelry, and ask her to lie down on her back. Kneel behind her head and apply a cleanser with smooth, outward strokes all over the face and neck, avoiding the eyes. Remove with damp cotton.

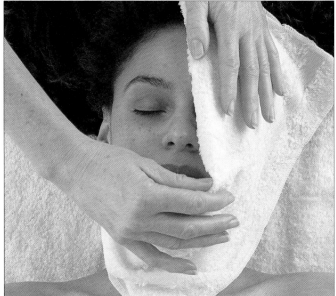

2 Soak three facecloths in a bowl of hot water containing a drop of essential oil or herbal tea bag (see above). Check the heat of the cloths, wring out, and cover the face (except the nose and mouth) with two cloths. As one cools, replace it. Blot dry.

BEGINNING TO MASSAGE

GENTLE MASSAGE OIL	JOJOBA CREAM	LUXURIOUS OIL

Essential oils
1 drop each of bergamot,
chamomile, and geranium
Carrier oil
10 ml sweet almond

Essential oil
4–6 drops of either jasmine,
frankincense, or lavender
Base
10 gm beeswax
25 ml sweet almond oil
20 ml sunflower oil, 35 ml jojoba
20 ml rosewater or distilled water

Essential oils
2 drops rose
1 drop each of jasmine and sandalwood
Carrier oils
5 ml each of apricot kernel oil and jojoba

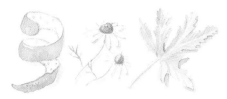

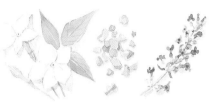

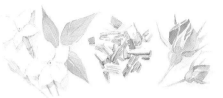

Follow method for basic oil, page 71.

Follow variation 1 for basic cream, page 72.

Follow method for basic oil, page 71.

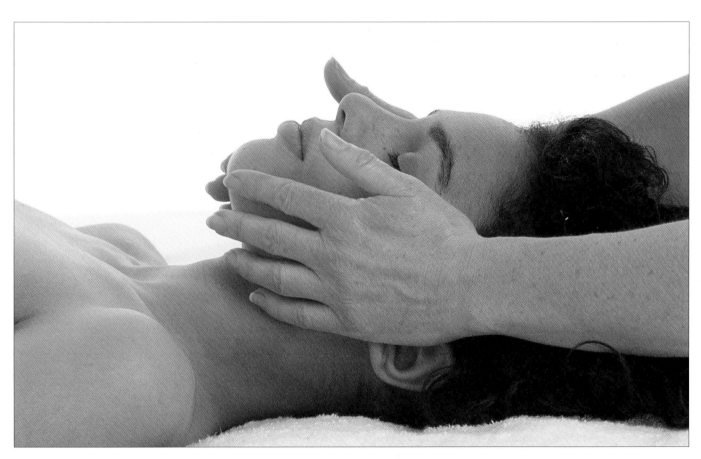

1 *Select an aromatic oil blend or cream to suit your friend (see above), and apply a small amount to your hands to warm it. Gently place your hands on the neck and stroke up to the chin.*

2 △ *Swivel your hands around at the chin to sweep out toward the ears. Imagine that you are sculpting the area, giving it a face-lift as your hands mold the contours.*

3 *Glide back gently to the chin where your fingers touch and interlock, then stroke your hands smoothly up over the cheeks and out to the temples.*

4 *At the temples, swivel your hands around so that your fingers meet over the forehead, and then stroke out over the forehead to the temples. Repeat steps 1–4 at least three times.*

RELEASING TENSION

1 Place the flattened fingers of both hands on the left side of the chest by the collarbone and stroke gently up to the neck at least six times. Then glide across the upper chest and repeat on the right side. If massaging a man, concentrate less on this stroking (stubble can make it uncomfortable for both of you) and more on circling and knuckling (steps 2 and 3).

2 Because so many people carry tension in the jaw, I do extra work here. Rest your left hand by your friend's left ear, and with the two middle fingers of your right hand make circles out from the chin along the left side of the jaw. Return to the chin and repeat on the right side.

3 ▷ Rotate the knuckles of both hands simultaneously on both sides of the face from under the cheek out to the jaw joints. Let each knuckle follow separately to produce a deep, steady movement.

4 With alternate hands, stroke around the chin and out along the jaw toward the ears in a rhythmic, sweeping movement. The more fluid you make this stroke, the more relaxing it will be. Repeat several times.

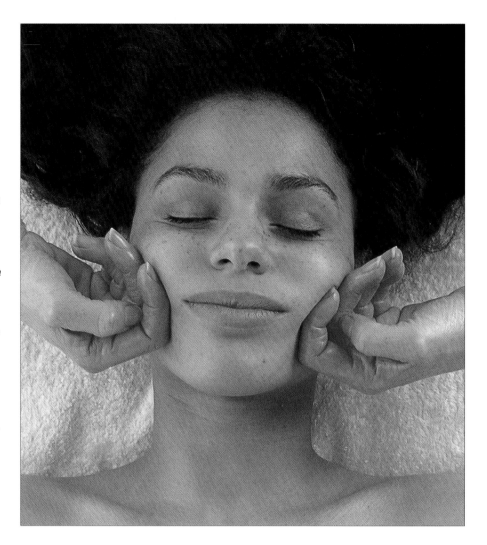

CIRCLING AWAY LINES

1 ▷ Interlock your thumbs in order to steady your hands, and with your middle fingers make circles all around the mouth and up the sides of the nose, taking care not to obstruct the nostrils. You can circle very gently or firmly — try both and ask your friend which movement she prefers.

2 Continue making circles, out from the center of the forehead to the right temple, varying the pressure as you work. Imagine lines and wrinkles disappearing as the nourishing oils penetrate the skin, helping to improve its texture, elasticity, and appearance. Repeat on the left side of the forehead.

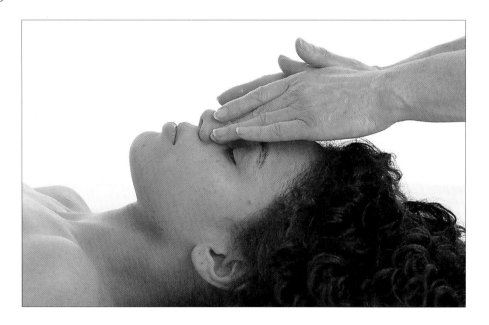

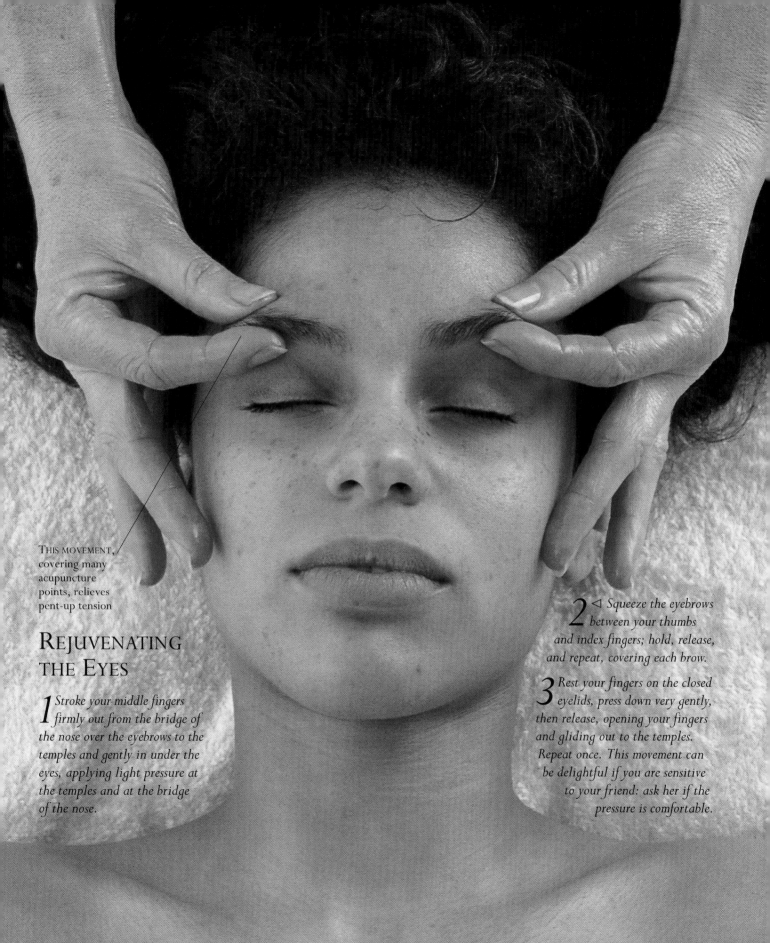

THIS MOVEMENT,
covering many
acupuncture
points, relieves
pent-up tension

REJUVENATING
THE EYES

1 Stroke your middle fingers firmly out from the bridge of the nose over the eyebrows to the temples and gently in under the eyes, applying light pressure at the temples and at the bridge of the nose.

2 ◁ Squeeze the eyebrows between your thumbs and index fingers; hold, release, and repeat, covering each brow.

3 Rest your fingers on the closed eyelids, press down very gently, then release, opening your fingers and gliding out to the temples. Repeat once. This movement can be delightful if you are sensitive to your friend: ask her if the pressure is comfortable.

RELAXING & SOOTHING

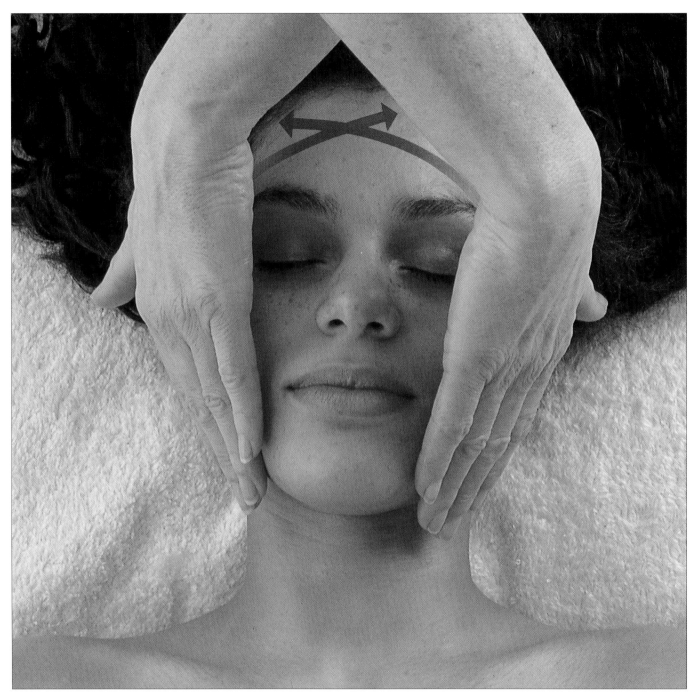

1 Stroke up the forehead, one hand slowly following the other. The very repetitiveness of this movement is its main virtue, allowing your friend to drift away.

2 With your fingertips, circle gently and continuously up from the bridge of the nose to the hairline. Then separate your fingers, slide them into the hair, and gently pull large sections of hair toward you. Work all over the head. This extraordinary movement creates a sensation of floating, as the last vestiges of tension melt away.

3 △ Stroke your palms out from the center of the forehead and glide down to the chin, where they cross (left hand lifts over right hand), return to the forehead and cross again. Glide your hands down the sides of the face and neck, swivel them out over the shoulders and up the back of the neck, then slide up the face to the forehead. Repeat two or three times.

4 Simply let your hands rest on your friend's forehead. Hold this position for at least ten seconds, and then slowly, imperceptibly, draw your hands away.

FINAL BEAUTIFYING TOUCHES

CLAY MASK

Essential oil
1 drop of either chamomile, geranium, or orange

Base
1 tsp fuller's earth, kaolin, or green clay
3 ml rosewater or distilled water
2 ml jojoba (optional, for dry skin)

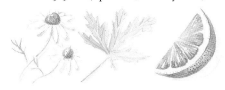

Follow variation 3 for basic clay mask, page 73.

MILD TONER

Essential oils
10 drops each of orange and petitgrain
5 drops neroli

Base
100 ml distilled water

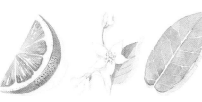

Follow method for basic toner, page 72.

GALEN'S ROSE CREAM

Essential oil
4 drops rose

Base
7 gm beeswax, 60 ml sweet almond oil
30 ml rosewater or distilled water

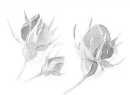

Follow method for basic cream, page 72.

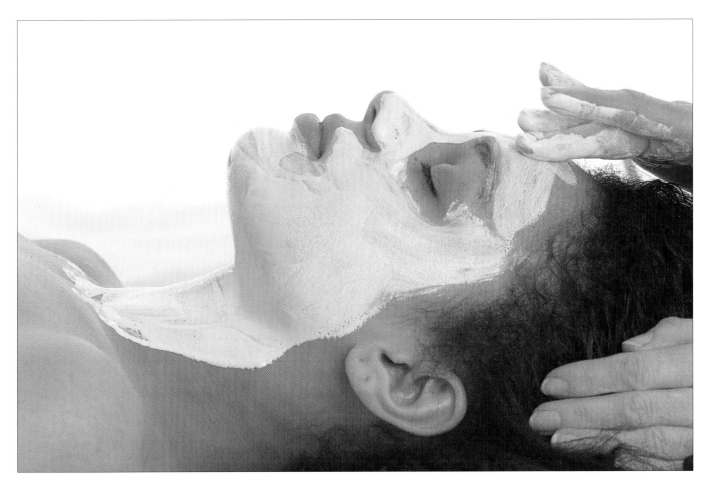

1 Remove the massage oil or cream with damp cotton, then clean your hands on a damp towel or facecloth.

2 △ Apply a clay mask all over the face and neck, avoiding the delicate eye area. Leave the mask to dry for about ten minutes, then remove it with a warm, damp facecloth.

3 Pour a small amount of toner on a piece of cotton, and gently stroke the entire face and neck with it. This helps to freshen the skin and remove any residue of the mask.

4 With your fingers, apply the moisturizing rose cream, which prevents moisture loss and keeps the skin smooth and pliable.

NATURAL FACE-LIFT

Taking ten minutes a day to massage your face can produce amazing results— simply relaxing tired, strained muscles can leave you looking ten years younger. Although wrinkles are an inevitable part of aging, massage can ease away microscopic lines so that your skin looks smoother and firmer, and it can help prevent new lines from appearing. Facial skin is delicate, so work gently using lots of scented oil that most suits your skin type (see page 71).

FOR OILY SKIN

Essential oils
2 drops bergamot
1 drop each of lemon and geranium
Carrier oil
10 ml soy

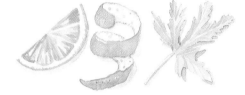

FOR SENSITIVE SKIN

Essential oils
2 drops chamomile, 1 drop lavender
Carrier oil
10 ml sweet almond

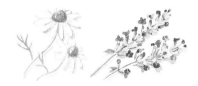

For all three recipes follow method for basic oil, page 71.

FOR DRY SKIN

Essential oils
2 drops neroli, 1 drop each of frankincense and rose
Carrier oils
5 ml each of sweet almond oil and jojoba

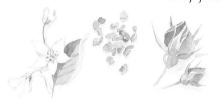

APPLYING THE OIL

Choose one of the massage oils and remove contact lenses and jewelry. Pour a small amount of the oil into your palm and warm it between your hands. Gently cup your face in your hands, and after a moment slide your hands out toward your ears, drawing tension out. Repeat at least three times.

FIRMING THE NECK & CHIN

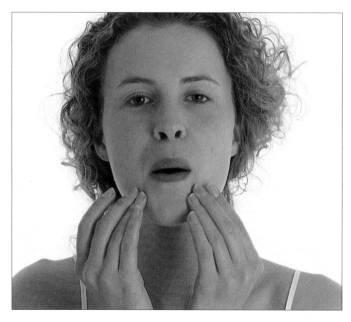

1 Open your mouth, pursing your lips tightly over your teeth to form an oval. Holding this position, make slow circular movements with the tips of your middle fingers around your mouth and chin and down to the edges of the jaw. Work up either side of the nose and out over the forehead to the temples.

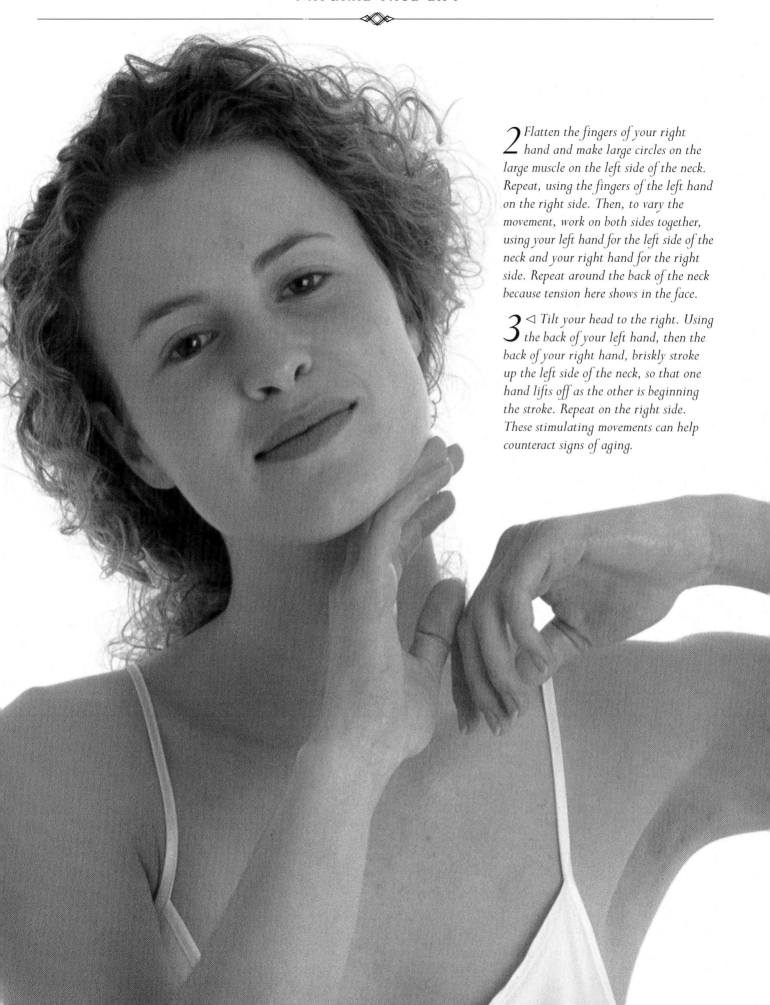

2 Flatten the fingers of your right
hand and make large circles on the
large muscle on the left side of the neck.
Repeat, using the fingers of the left hand
on the right side. Then, to vary the
movement, work on both sides together,
using your left hand for the left side of the
neck and your right hand for the right
side. Repeat around the back of the neck
because tension here shows in the face.

3 ◁ Tilt your head to the right. Using
the back of your left hand, then the
back of your right hand, briskly stroke
up the left side of the neck, so that one
hand lifts off as the other is beginning
the stroke. Repeat on the right side.
These stimulating movements can help
counteract signs of aging.

BEAUTIFYING THE EYES

1 With your two middle fingers circle your eyes, stroking firmly out over the eyebrows and gliding very gently back under the eyes. Repeat five times.

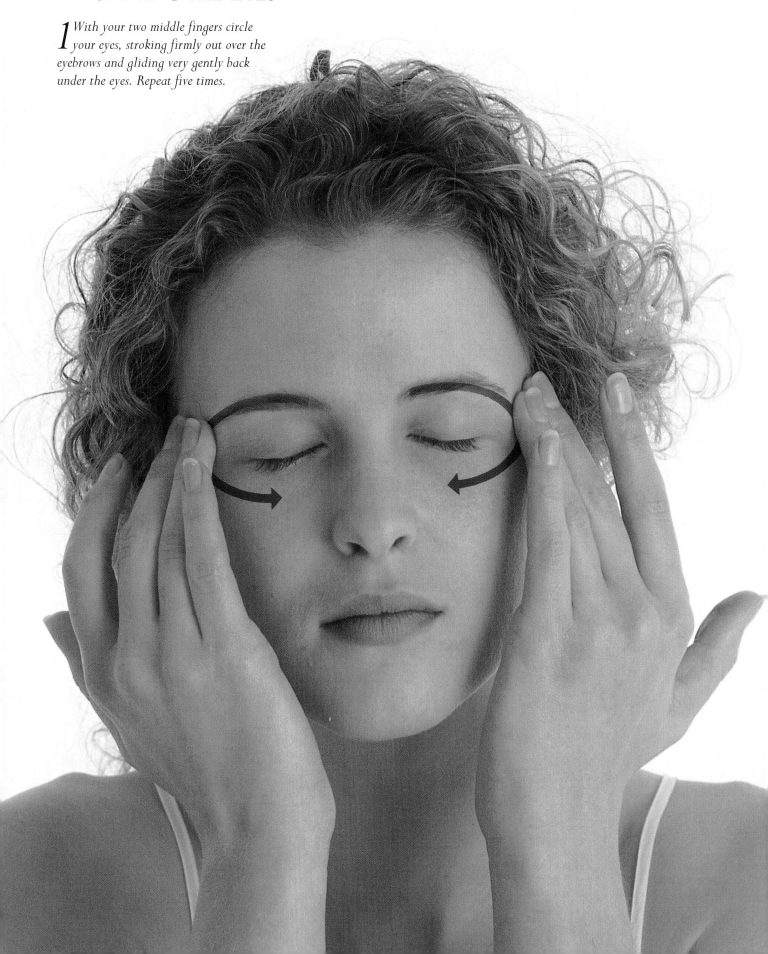

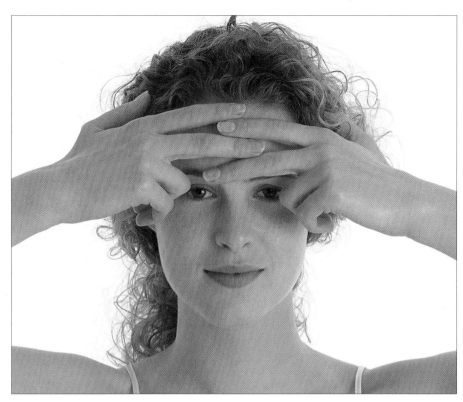

2 Starting at the bridge of the nose, squeeze the eyebrows between your thumbs and first two fingers. Hold, and slowly release before moving on to the next area, covering the whole eyebrow.

3 Apply pressure with the middle fingers of both hands on the temples and all over the forehead. This can help relieve headaches and tension. Then use just your third fingers to apply gentle pressure along the socket bone beneath the eyes, in the direction of the nose.

4 ◁ Combat frown lines by rubbing your fingers together in a scissor-like motion across the middle of the forehead, above the eyebrows, and out to each side of the forehead.

5 Slowly stroke one palm after the other from the eyebrows over the forehead and into the hair. Repeat several times.

GENTLE REVITALIZATION

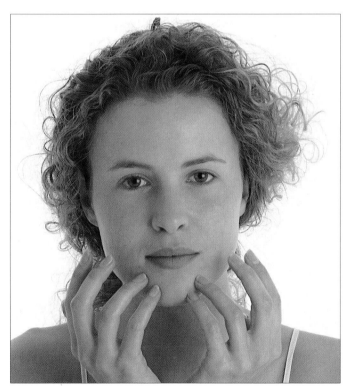

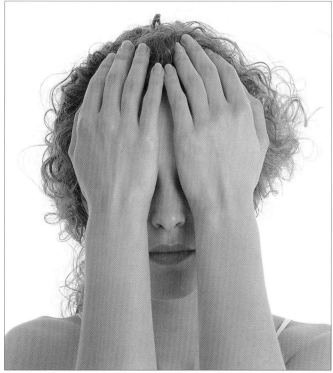

1 With your fingertips, lightly tap from the chin out to the ears, then from beside the nose up to the temples and, finally, over the forehead to the temples. Tap extremely gently over the closed eyelid and beneath the eye (remove contact lenses first).

2 Enjoy the quietness and stillness of just cupping your hands over your eyes and forehead to release any last vestiges of tension. Alternatively, cup your hands over the whole face, including the chin and cheeks. Hold for several seconds.

REFRESHING FACIAL

The brisk and energetic movements in this invigorating facial massage stimulate the circulation, bringing fresh, oxygenated blood to the area and eliminating waste to leave the skin glowing. Surprisingly, vigorous strokes can be deeply relaxing and are an essential part of this facial massage. Skin toners are used to freshen the skin, remove traces of cleanser and help restore the skin's acid mantle (a fine layer that protects against infection). They can also be used after a refreshing facial for a cooling effect. A simple splash of water is the cheapest skin toner, but traditional preparations include flower waters, herbal infusions, and aromatic vinegars. To preserve the natural equilibrium of the skin, I recommend mild skin fresheners.

GENTLE ROSE TONER

Essential oil
25 drops rose
Base
100 ml distilled water

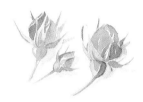

Follow method for basic toner, page 72.

HONEY WATER

Essential oils
2 drops bergamot, 1 drop each of lavender, sandalwood, and benzoin
Base
10 ml vodka
¼ tsp honey
80 ml orange flower water

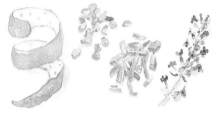

Follow method for basic honey water, page 72.

AROMATIC VINEGAR

Essential oils
3 drops rosemary
2 drops rose, 1 drop lavender
Base
10 ml wine or cider vinegar
80 ml distilled water

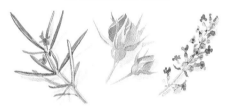

Follow method for basic aromatic vinegar, page 72.

TONING THE CHIN

1 ▷ Choose one of the aromatic toners above and pour a small amount in your palm. Splash the toner on your face, taking care to avoid the eyes. Then, with the backs of your hands, rhythmically slap and pat the area under the chin. Repeat several times. This movement can help combat a double chin by stimulating the circulation.

2 Loosely roll the backs of your fingers under the chin, one hand following the other. Vary the amount of pressure from a light, vibrating movement to a firm, invigorating one. Continue on the left and right sides of the chin.

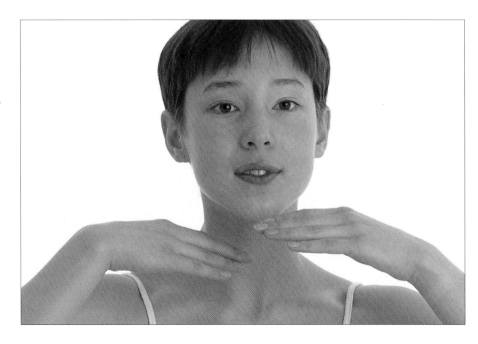

RESISTING THE EFFECTS OF AGING

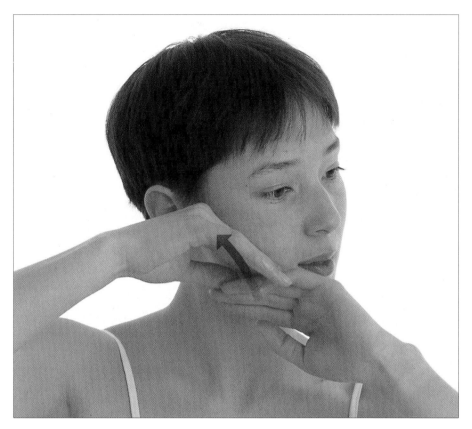

1 ◁ *Roll the skin of the right cheek with the backs of all your fingers from the right side of the mouth over the cheek toward the ear. Both hands work together, one following the other. Work upward and outward, following the facial muscles. This will improve tone and give sagging cheeks a boost. Repeat on the left side.*

2 *Ease frown lines by tapping the fleshy part of your fingers rapidly up the forehead. This percussive movement sounds like galloping horses.*

3 *Using your fingertips, lightly and rhythmically tap all over the face. Some clients say this feels like butterfly wings fluttering on the face while others claim it is like raindrops falling. On a hot day, splash some extra toner on the face and pat it in using this stimulating movement to leave the skin fresh and glowing. Some men like to do this refreshing movement after shaving.*

INSTANT REVIVAL

1 ▷ *Starting at the bridge of your nose, make circular movements with the pads of your fingers in a straight line up to the top of your head. Then work firmly and methodically all over your head, really moving the scalp as if you were shampooing your hair. This invigorating action helps release tension and stimulate the circulation, and can also relieve headaches.*

2 *With your fingers against the scalp, take large handfuls of hair and gently yet firmly pull up at the roots.*

3 *Finish the refreshing facial by using your thumbs and forefingers to massage your ears. Begin at the lobes and squeeze, rotate, and release, working up to the top of the ear. Acupuncture points relating to the whole body are found on the ears and massaging these points stimulates every part of you.*

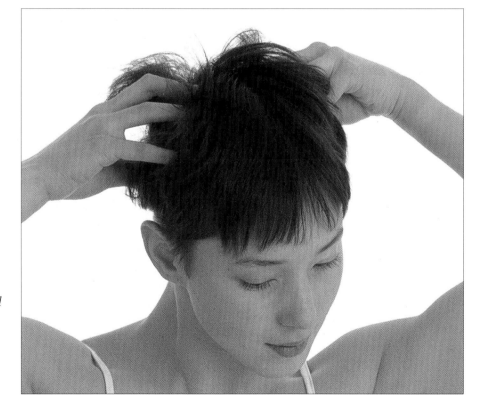

BEAUTIFYING THE BODY

Everybody should learn how to do simple self-massage because it is an excellent way to pamper yourself, and when combined with essential oils, it is remarkably beneficial. In just a few minutes each day, you can improve both the condition and the tone of your skin. Choose aromatic oils to suit your needs – to cleanse, stimulate, or nourish – and, most important, choose an oil blend with a scent that you find personally appealing.

HANDS & ELBOWS

THE CONDITION OF THE HANDS and elbows depends largely on the care we give them. Age, hard work, and neglect can leave them rough and dry, while water and detergents strip away protective oils. For smoother hands, massage in a nourishing cream containing a soothing oil, such as benzoin. Cover dry hands with extra rich cream at night and wear cotton gloves to bed, as did ladies of the court in Elizabethan England.

NOURISHING THE HANDS

1 Sit comfortably and apply a little cream (see opposite page) to your right palm. Stroke it on your left hand from the fingers to the wrist. Imagine the cream penetrating the skin – relaxing, soothing, and warming it. Repeat several times.

2 ▷ Supporting your left palm with the fingers of your right hand, use your thumb to stroke from the knuckle of your little finger down the tendon toward the wrist. Repeat, stroking down the tendons between each of the fingers.

3 Squeeze the base of your little finger between your thumb and forefinger and circle around either side of the finger, working up to and including the tip of the nail. Rub some cream into the cuticle and fingernail, which also benefit from pampering. Repeat on each finger and on the thumb.

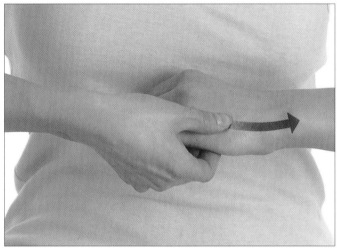

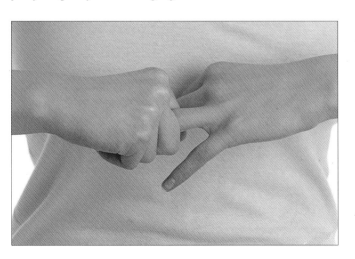

4 ◁ Using the knuckles of the first and second fingers, gently grip the little finger and slowly pull it as you slide up to the tip with a corkscrew-like motion that stimulates the circulation. Repeat twice on each finger and on the thumb.

5 Support the back of the left hand with the fingers of your right hand and massage the palm with your thumb. Stroke and stretch the palm and notice tension melting away.

6 Firmly roll your middle knuckles all over the palm and finish by gently stroking the wrist, and then the hand, with your thumb. Repeat the entire sequence on the other hand.

PAMPERING THE ELBOWS

With care and attention, you can transform rough, dry and discolored elbows. For a gentle bleaching effect, rub each elbow with half a lemon, and to reverse dryness, massage elbows with a generous amount of one of these rich creams, containing nourishing oils such as avocado and wheatgerm.

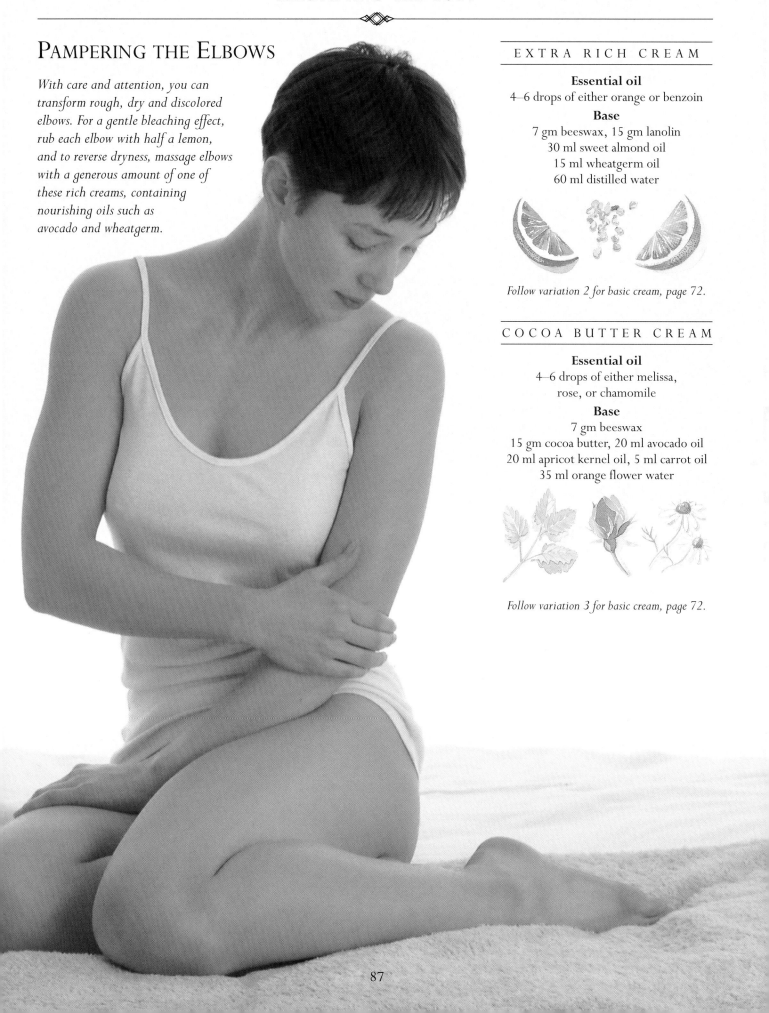

EXTRA RICH CREAM

Essential oil
4–6 drops of either orange or benzoin

Base
7 gm beeswax, 15 gm lanolin
30 ml sweet almond oil
15 ml wheatgerm oil
60 ml distilled water

Follow variation 2 for basic cream, page 72.

COCOA BUTTER CREAM

Essential oil
4–6 drops of either melissa,
rose, or chamomile

Base
7 gm beeswax
15 gm cocoa butter, 20 ml avocado oil
20 ml apricot kernel oil, 5 ml carrot oil
35 ml orange flower water

Follow variation 3 for basic cream, page 72.

ABDOMEN, HIPS & THIGHS

MANY OF MY CLIENTS wish to transform these fleshy, untoned areas, which are prone to cellulite (dimpled flesh resembling orange peel, caused by connective tissue pulling in against the skin, making the fat bulge). Daily aromatherapy massage can improve the skin by making it appear smoother and tighter to give the illusion of lost weight. Large, firm movements boost the circulation and soft, smooth strokes stimulate the lymphatic system. Beneficial essential oils include: marjoram and peppermint to soothe the abdomen; rosemary and geranium to invigorate; and juniper to help reduce fluid retention.

SOOTHING BLEND

Essential oils
3 drops marjoram, 2 drops chamomile
1 drop peppermint
Carrier oils
18 ml sweet almond, 2 ml wheatgerm

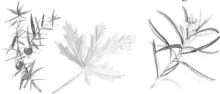

CELLULITE BLEND

Essential oils
3 drops each of lavender and cypress
1 drop juniper
Carrier oils
18 ml sweet almond, 2 ml wheatgerm

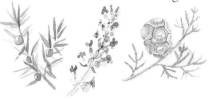

STIMULATING BLEND

Essential oils
3 drops each of juniper and rosemary
1 drop geranium
Carrier oils
18 ml sweet almond, 2 ml wheatgerm

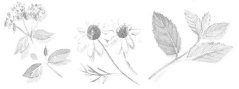

For all, follow method for basic oil, page 71.

IMPROVING THE ABDOMEN & HIPS

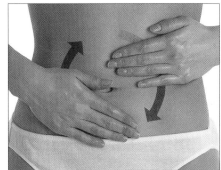

1 Sit comfortably and rest your left hand on your diaphragm (just under the rib cage) while your right hand applies about a teaspoon of oil with clockwise strokes around the navel (following the workings of the intestine). Now introduce the left hand to the stroke so that both hands circle the navel (see Circular Stroking, page 45). Repeat several times.

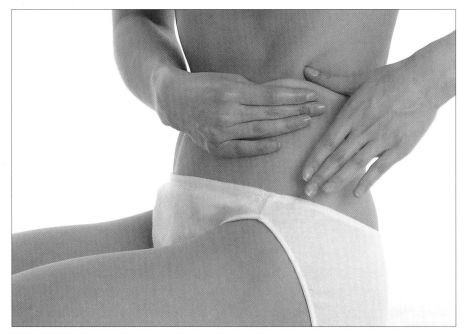

2 △ Knead the hips, waist, and abdomen by squeezing and lifting the flesh with one hand and releasing it into the other. Knead all over this area, wherever you can pick up enough flesh.

3 With your left hand on top of your right, use your fingertips to apply gentle circular pressure all around the navel. Work in a clockwise direction.

4 Finish by gently stroking all over the abdomen and hips. This is soothing and stimulates the lymphatic system.

TONING THE THIGHS

1 Apply more massage oil if necessary so that your hands move smoothly over the skin. Gently stroke up from your left knee, directing your movements toward the inner thigh. Then stroke from the back of the knee up to the buttocks.

4 Place your left hand on the back of the outer thigh and your right hand on the back of the inner thigh. Pull the flesh up to the top of the thigh, release, and cross your hands down the other side. Repeat this crisscross movement several times.

5 Stroke smoothly and gently from above the knee to the top of the thigh and from the back of the knee to the buttock. This repetitive stroking stimulates the lymphatic system. Repeat the sequence on the right thigh.

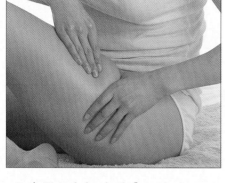

2 △ Knead the thigh from the knee up to the top of the leg. This area is fleshy, so use deep movements to squeeze and lift the flesh. These kneading strokes stimulate the circulation and break down dimpled skin by helping stored fluid and waste to be reabsorbed into the lymphatic system. Repeat on the back of the thigh.

3 ▷ Applying firm pressure, rotate the knuckles of both hands all over the front and back of the thigh.

THE FEET

LEONARDO DA VINCI referred to the foot as the world's greatest engineering device: it contains nearly a quarter of the body's bones and absorbs three times the body's weight with each step. Yet the feet are often neglected. Tired, aching feet affect the way you look, feel and move. Each foot contains thousands of nerve endings, and regular massage benefits the whole body while keeping the feet smooth and flexible. For a pre-massage treat, soak the feet in a tub of warm water containing four drops of essential oil: juniper, lemongrass, or rosemary to combat fluid retention; cypress or geranium for cramps; or eucalyptus to revitalize.

TIRED FEET BLEND

Essential oil
4 drops of either lavender or peppermint
Carrier oil
10 ml sunflower or sweet almond

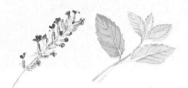

Follow method for basic oil, page 71.

POMADE FOR ROUGH SKIN

Essential oil
20 drops of either frankincense, geranium, or sandalwood
Base
15 gm beeswax
100 ml sunflower or sweet almond oil

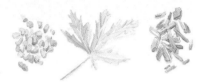

Follow method for basic pomade, page 73.

SWOLLEN FEET BLEND

Essential oils
3 drops lavender, 2 drops chamomile
Carrier oil
10 ml sunflower or sweet almond

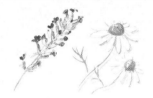

Follow method for basic oil, page 71.

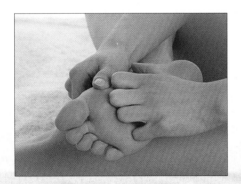

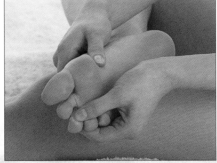

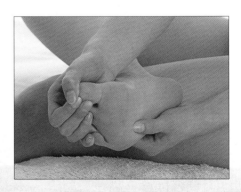

1 Rest your right foot on your left thigh. Support it with your right hand while your left hand strokes the sole and top of the foot from the toes up to the ankle, spreading the aromatic oil or pomade. Use your knuckles to ripple all around the sole. Then, using your thumbs, apply deep pressure to the sole of the foot (see Static Pressures, page 46). Work on the center, outer side, and instep.

2 Massage each toe by rubbing, squeezing, and gently rolling it between your fingers. Then pinch the tip of the nail. These movements stimulate the circulation and soothe the toes.

3 Support your foot with your left hand, and clasp your toes with the right hand. Gently stretch the toes backward and forward to release tension and increase their flexibility.

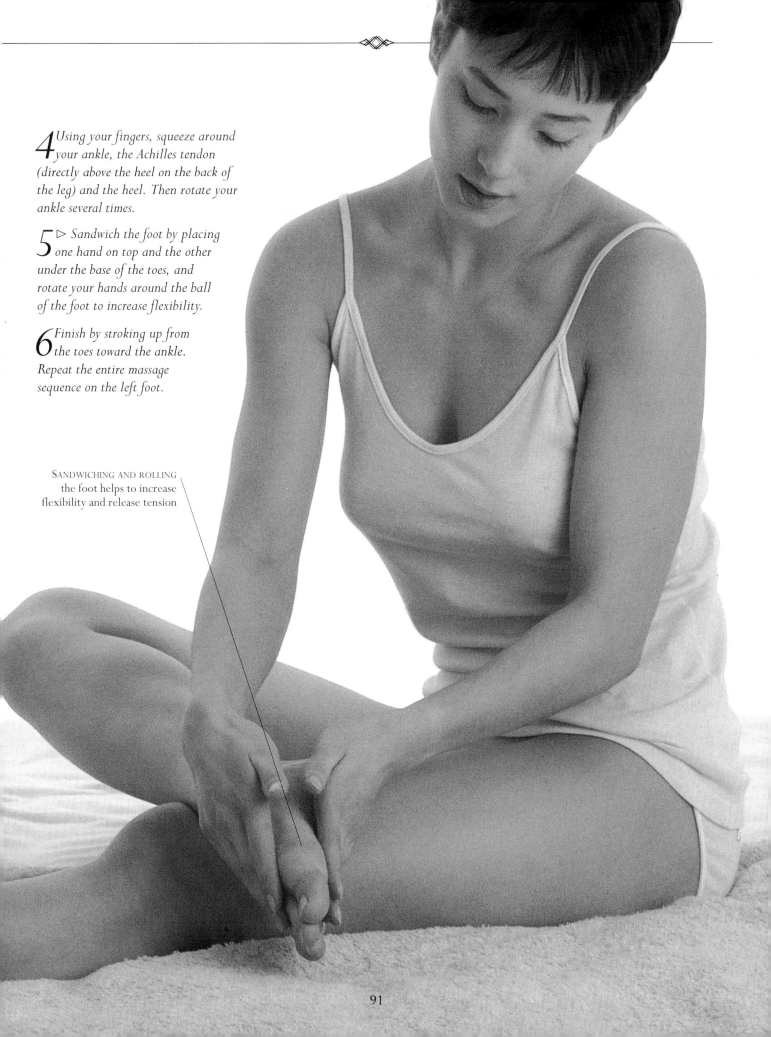

4 Using your fingers, squeeze around your ankle, the Achilles tendon (directly above the heel on the back of the leg) and the heel. Then rotate your ankle several times.

5 ▷ Sandwich the foot by placing one hand on top and the other under the base of the toes, and rotate your hands around the ball of the foot to increase flexibility.

6 Finish by stroking up from the toes toward the ankle. Repeat the entire massage sequence on the left foot.

SANDWICHING AND ROLLING the foot helps to increase flexibility and release tension

SCENTED BATHING

A fragranced bath, whether warming and comforting or coolly refreshing, has always been recognized as the perfect way to shed tension. The Greek physician Hippocrates (*c.*460 – 377BC) maintained that "the way to health is to have an aromatic bath and scented massage every day." Most famous beauties have had extravagant bath recipes, containing ingredients such as crushed strawberries and champagne, but the simple addition of diluted essential oils can make a bath equally luxurious. If you do not have a bath, an aromatherapy shower also works wonders.

EXTRAVAGANT BLEND

Essential oils
2 drops each of neroli and rose
1 drop sandalwood
Carrier oil
5 ml sweet almond

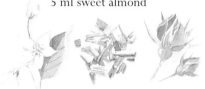

Follow method for basic oil, page 71.

MILK & HONEY BATH

Essential oil
10-25 drops of mandarin or geranium
Base
1 tsp liquid detergent
110 ml of either sweet almond
or sunflower oil
25 ml vodka
55 ml milk
1 tsp honey
1 egg

Makes enough for eight baths. Mix the ingredients in a blender on low speed.

WAKE-UP BLEND

Essential oils
2 drops each of petitgrain and rosemary
1 drop geranium
Carrier oil
5 ml sweet almond

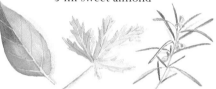

Follow method for basic oil, page 71.

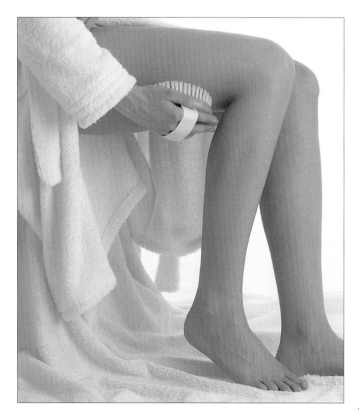

SKIN BRUSHING

◁ *Before you climb into your scented bath or step into the shower, take a few minutes to stimulate the circulation by brushing your skin with a natural fiber skin brush or glove. Use brisk, circular movements all over the body, bringing fresh blood to the surface, removing dead cells, and unclogging pores.*

PREPARING THE BATH

While the bath is filling with warm water (avoid very hot water, which strips the skin of natural oils, thereby drying it out), dilute up to 5 drops of your chosen essential oils in the carrier oil. Add the oil blend when the bath is nearly full, so you can enjoy the effects fully before the oils begin to evaporate. To enhance the relaxing atmosphere, bathe by candlelight.

FRAGRANT SHOWERING

If you prefer a shower to a bath, you can still enjoy the benefits of aromatherapy by dissolving 12 drops of up to three of your favorite essential oils in 30 ml liquid soap.

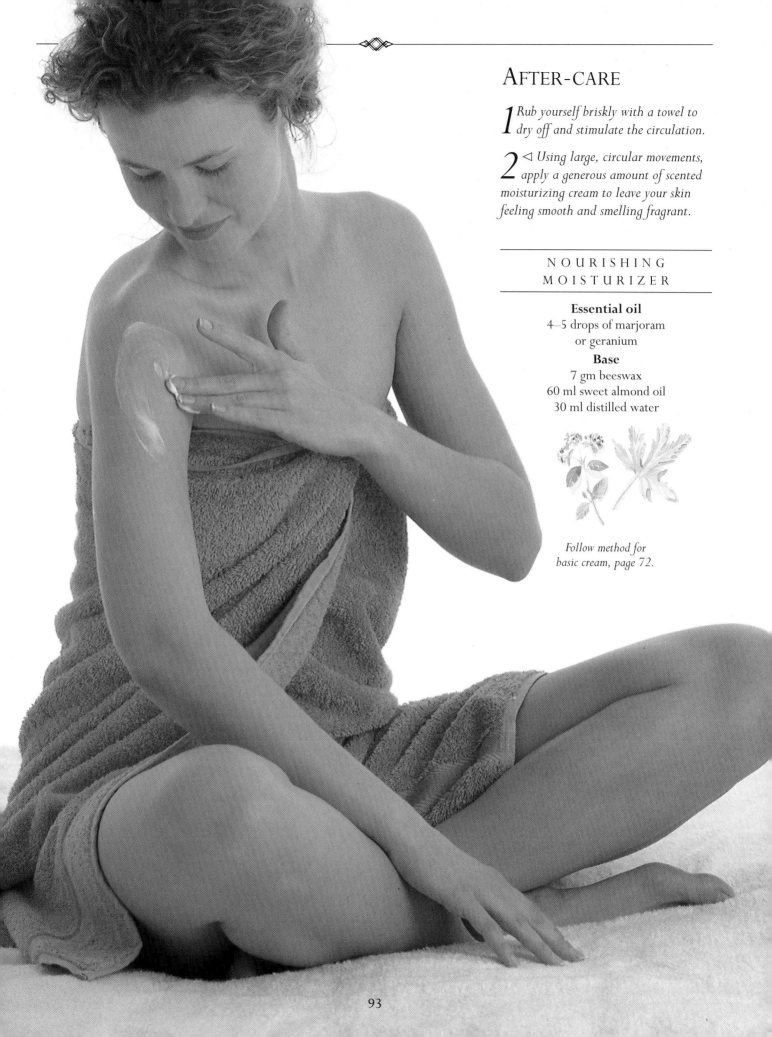

AFTER-CARE

1 Rub yourself briskly with a towel to dry off and stimulate the circulation.

2 ◁ Using large, circular movements, apply a generous amount of scented moisturizing cream to leave your skin feeling smooth and smelling fragrant.

NOURISHING MOISTURIZER

Essential oil
4–5 drops of marjoram
or geranium
Base
7 gm beeswax
60 ml sweet almond oil
30 ml distilled water

*Follow method for
basic cream, page 72.*

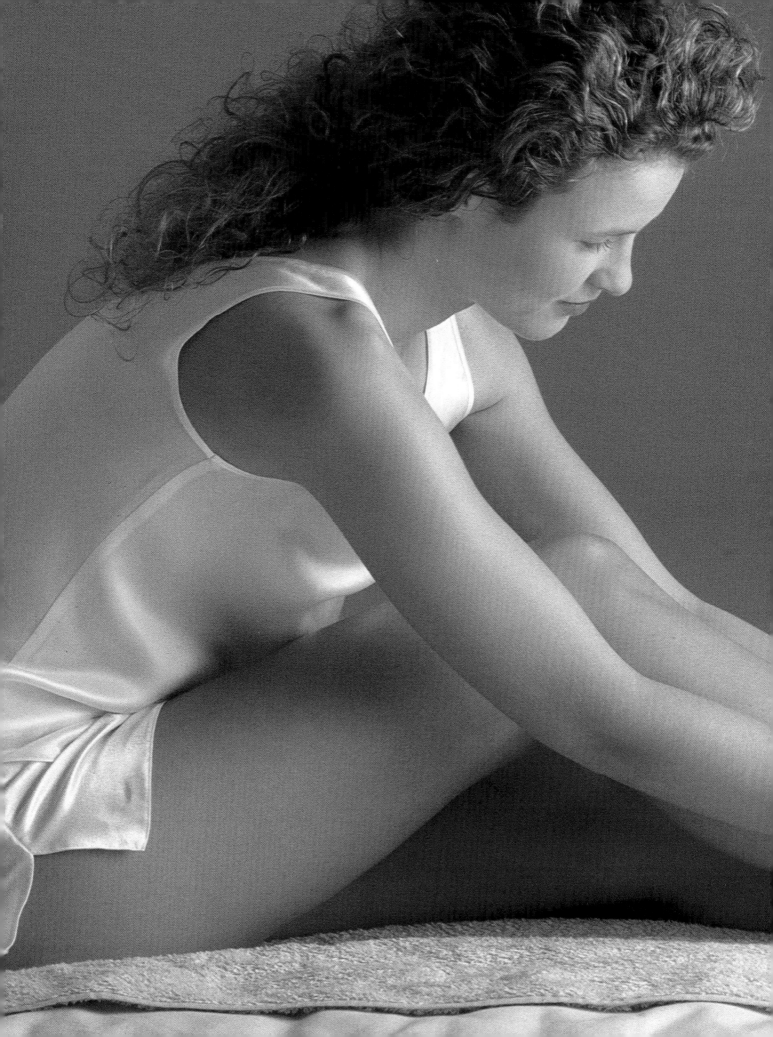

THERAPEUTIC REMEDIES

*Essential oils have strong healing properties.
Inhaling a few drops of eucalyptus oil, for example,
clears congestion, and adding lavender oil to a relaxing
bath promotes sleep, while massage with rosemary oil
eases aches and pains. The sheer pleasure of massage
is therapeutic, and, when combined with aromatic oils,
the healing effect is even more profound.*

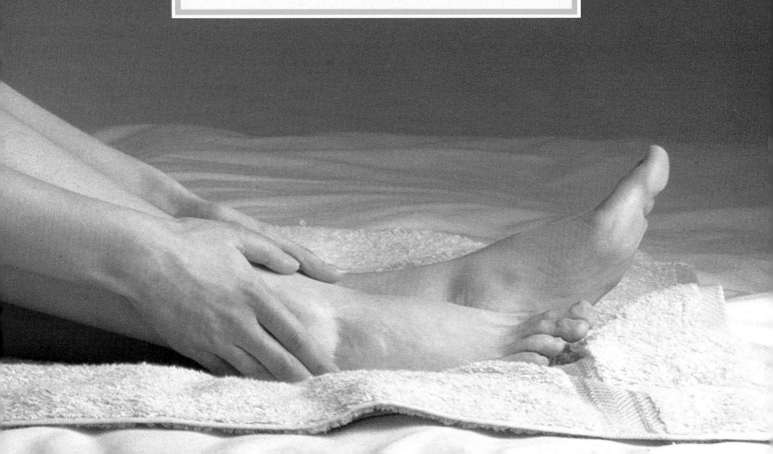

AROMATHERAPY & HEALTH

Whether we are young or old, healthy and at the peak of physical fitness or frail and infirm, the complementary therapies of aromatherapy and massage can enhance our lives and help prevent illness. By awakening the senses of smell and touch, we can relieve tension, improve sleep, enhance mood, and alleviate many physical ailments. Above all, they impart a sense of well-being so important to overall health. Medical research has shown there is indeed a strong connection between positive mood and good health.

THE BENEFITS OF FRAGRANCE

Out of all five senses, smell has the most direct connection to the emotional center of the brain, and there is increasing evidence to prove the physiological and psychological benefits of fragrance. Odors are first detected in the nasal mucosa located behind the bridge of the nose, and containing millions of olfactory receptor cells. When we inhale, odor molecules are filtered and warmed and stimulate the olfactory neurons (nerve cells). Information then travels to the limbic section of the brain, the part associated with memories, feelings, arousal, and emotion.

Clinical and laboratory research conducted by Susan Schiffman of Duke University's Department of Psychology in Durham, North Carolina has shown that certain scents promote relaxation, reduce stress, and alleviate depression, while others increase memory retrieval, help improve self-image, enhance sexuality, or modify sleep patterns. Her research has included studies in which patients have been taught relaxation techniques and, when fully relaxed, have had an odor placed under their nostrils. With repetition, the patient begins to associate the odor with relaxation, and in time, the odor alone will provoke the relaxation response. Schiffman has also found that certain odors, such as lavender and neroli, may induce relaxation in a patient with no previous conditioning. I believe this work to be of interest to anyone practicing massage with aromatic oils, because it reveals the potential benefits of this treatment for stress-related problems.

FEELING GOOD TO STAY HEALTHY

Studies have shown that people who live with high levels of stress are less resistant to illness and disease than those with low stress levels. In 1991 at Carnegie Mellon University in Pittsburgh, Pennsylvania, researchers gave 394 healthy people a questionnaire assessing their levels of stress, then exposed them to cold viruses. Almost half of those who described their stress levels as high caught the cold, compared with only a quarter of those who described their stress levels as low. The medical profession has long suspected that there is a strong link between stress and illness. High blood pressure and heart disease, for example, are thought to be stress-related, and even cancer, arthritis, and infertility have been shown to have a higher occurrence rate when stress is high.

Happily, the reverse is also true. In another study carried out in 1987, researchers analyzed saliva and found that the immune system of those participating was functioning at a higher level when they were in a positive mood than when they were in a negative mood. Since the immune system helps the body defend itself against infections, this demonstrates that feeling good really does have a beneficial effect on one's ability to stay healthy. Massage with essential oils is a wonderful way to relax the body and mind and increase positive outlook, thus relieving stress, preventing illness, and enhancing quality of life.

RELIEVING PAIN

Massage, both with aromatic oils and without, is used extensively in hospitals throughout Europe, especially in Britain, and in Australia and South Africa. At the hospitals and at the Royal College of Nursing in London where I teach, nurses find that massage helps patients enormously. It is a very physical way of showing care and concern. It also aids relaxation and reduces pain, relieving anxiety and improving sleep. Touch and massage are forms of communication that help nurses understand and make personal contact with their patients. When essential oils are used, the delightful aromas soon transform a drab clinical ward into a room with a fragrant, friendly atmosphere.

It is rewarding to see how even the simplest of treatments – a foot or hand massage – can have such a profound effect, bringing comfort, sympathy, and reassurance – the perfect complement to medication. As one client said, "Massage really eased my pain, and the scent calmed me down, reminding me of my garden and of happier and healthier times. It was the turning point of my recovery." But you do not have to be ill or in the hospital to benefit from the therapeutic effects of massage and aromatherapy. Everyone can benefit by enhancing the home or workplace with aromatic essential oils.

HEALING WITH OILS

Essential oils can be used to treat a range of ailments. Some benefit from massage with aromatic oils, while others respond best to the oils alone – guidelines are given below for other applications. The charts on the following pages will guide you in using appropriate oils. Each chart is accompanied by three especially useful recipes for common complaints, but for other ailments follow the directions in the chart. For **Massage Blends** or **Other Applications**, choose from up to four of the **Useful Essential Oils** by selecting those with scents that appeal to you. Combine the recommended number of drops with a carrier oil to suit your skin type (see page 14), following the blending guide on page 15. These remedies have been effective on many people, but if your condition does not improve within one or two days, visit a doctor, and seek professional advice for any persistent condition.

OTHER WAYS TO USE ESSENTIAL OILS

—— IN COMPRESSES ——
Use warm compresses to ease backache or abdominal pains; cold compresses for treating headaches, swollen joints, bruises, and sprains. Add up to 6 drops of essential oil to a large bowl of water (hot for warm compresses, cold for cold compresses). Stir, then place a facecloth on the water's surface to collect a film of oil. Wring out and apply to the affected area for 10–20 minutes, resoaking the cloth as needed to maintain its temperature.

—— AS INHALATIONS ——
& FACIAL STEAMS
Inhalations are invaluable for easing respiratory problems, phlegm, sore throats, and coughs, and are an effective way to open the pores to deep-cleanse the skin. Do not use inhalations if you have asthma or broken capillaries. Fill a large bowl

with boiling water and add 2–6 drops of essential oil. Lean over the bowl and, if you wish, cover your head with a towel to trap the steam for five to ten minutes – take deep breaths and shut your eyes since the vapor from the oils can sting. For skin problems, do not use more than once a week; for respiratory problems, use up to three times a day.

—— AS AIR FRESHENERS ——
To keep away insects, rid the air of cooking smells, and generally freshen up the home, add 5 drops of essential oil to 1 cup of cooled, boiled water in a plant sprayer. Shake well, and spray the room. Lemongrass and lavender are among my favorite air-freshening scents.

—— IN VAPORIZERS ——
A range of essential oil burners made from clay are available from health stores. Usually, a small candle is lit

below a bowl containing 2–4 drops of essential oil added to water. The candle's heat warms the bowl, and the essential oils evaporate, scenting the room. Do not let the water evaporate completely, since the bowl may crack. Keep away from children.

—— TO SCENT FLOORS ——
& WORK SURFACES
To scent floors, add 2 drops of essential oil to the water before mopping the area. Use any of your favorite oils. I find rosemary, lemongrass and lemon beautifully fresh. Scrubbing kitchen surfaces with essential oils can disinfect as well as scent. Eucalyptus oil is probably the best-known disinfectant. Add 2 drops to 100 ml water, before wiping. If you find the scent of eucalyptus too medicinal, try lavender, lemon, or pine.

STRESS

WE ALL NEED A CERTAIN AMOUNT of stress to add zest and excitement to our lives, but too much can damage our health. Excessive stress can lead to minor ailments, such as headaches and stomachaches, but if it persists it can cause more serious problems. Even heart attacks and cancer are thought more likely to occur in those whose resistance is low. It is not necessarily the stress that causes illness, but how we react to and deal with

it. To cope with stress, we need to learn to recognize our own limitations and be aware of our levels of anxiety or physical exhaustion. Massage can help us to do this and is also an excellent way to teach people what it feels like to be relaxed. To make a massage oil blend, choose up to four of your favorite essential oils from those suggested and blend with a carrier oil to suit your skin type (see page 14).

Choose either German or Roman chamomile (see page 19).

PROBLEM	USEFUL ESSENTIAL OILS		GENERAL EFFECT OF OILS
INSOMNIA Including difficulty in going to sleep and staying asleep, or simply trouble relaxing and releasing the day's tension.	*Chamomile Lavender Marjoram Neroli Orange	Petitgrain	Sedative, calming, tension-relieving oils help relaxation.
MENTAL FATIGUE OR NERVOUS EXHAUSTION When the mind feels exhausted from long periods of concentration.	Clary sage Lemongrass Mandarin Peppermint Rosemary		Invigorating oils help wake up the body, stimulate the mind, and aid concentration.
LACK OF CONFIDENCE Including feeling nervous or anxious and in need of reassurance.	Bergamot *Chamomile Clary sage Jasmine	Mandarin Orange Rose Sandalwood	Stimulating, refreshing, and exotic oils help boost confidence.
DEPRESSION & LETHARGY Including lack of energy, vitality, and positive feelings, hopelessness, melancholy, and lack of interest.	Bergamot Clary sage Geranium Jasmine Lavender	Melissa Orange Sandalwood	Oils with beautiful aromas lift the spirits, promote a sense of well-being, and help revive the body and mind when energy is lacking.
STRESS Including feeling tense, anxious, and unable to unwind resulting from great demands on physical and mental energy.	*Chamomile Frankincense Juniper Lavender Lemongrass	Marjoram Neroli Orange Petitgrain Sandalwood	Soothing oils with a calming and sedative effect help relax the mind.
JET LAG When the body and mind need calming in order to sleep or, alternatively, when the traveler needs to feel alert and uplifted to minimize the effects of crossing time zones.	CALMING Clary sage Geranium Lavender Petitgrain Rose	UPLIFTING Bergamot Melissa Orange Peppermint Rosemary	Oils with familiar scents help regulate sleep patterns; or stimulating oils help keep the body awake and the mind alert.

TO EASE STRESS	TO PROMOTE SLEEP	TO UPLIFT
Essential oils	**Essential oils**	**Essential oils**
5 drops sandalwood	4 drops lavender, 2 drops each of	4 drops bergamot
2 drops each of neroli and clary sage	Roman chamomile and neroli	2 drops geranium
Carrier oil	**Carrier oil**	1 drop melissa
20 ml sweet almond	20 ml sweet almond	**Carrier oil**
		20 ml sweet almond

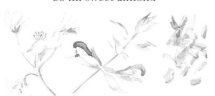

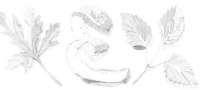

For all three recipes, follow method for basic oil, page 71.

MASSAGE BLEND	**MASSAGE TREATMENT**	**OTHER APPLICATIONS**
Add up to 8 drops essential oils to 20 ml carrier oil.	A slow, rhythmic back massage followed by cat stroking (see page 47) has a hypnotic effect and lulls the person being massaged to sleep.	• *Place 2–4 drops of essential oils on the pillow to encourage sleep.* • *Add up to 5 drops of essential oils to the bath (single oils or combinations of two) – using the same oil blend as for the massage reinforces the sedative message.*
Add up to 8 drops essential oils to 20 ml carrier oil.	Circular pressures (see page 46) over the forehead, temples, and scalp, followed by a scalp massage (see page 85) to stimulate the circulation.	• *Use 4 drops of essential oils in a vaporizer (see page 97) or add 5 drops of essential oils to 1 cup of water to make an air freshener (see page 97).* • *Use 4 drops of essential oil in an inhalation (see page 97).* **Do not use if you have asthma**.
Add up to 8 drops essential oils to 20 ml carrier oil.	A full body massage (see pages 48–67), concentrating on any particular areas of tension or a stimulating scalp massage (see page 85).	• *Add up to 5 drops of essential oils to the bath.*
Add up to 8 drops essential oils to 20 ml carrier oil.	Start with a full body massage (see pages 48–67) to boost vitality. Follow with an energizing foot massage (see pages 90–1) or a stimulating scalp massage (see page 85).	• *Add up to 5 drops of essential oils to the bath.*
Add up to 8 drops essential oils to 20 ml carrier oil.	A full body massage (see pages 48–67) focusing on slow, rhythmic strokes to help calm, followed by smooth strokes on the shoulders, neck, and face (see pages 56–9).	• *Add up to 5 drops of essential oils to the bath.*
To aid sleep: add up to 8 drops calming essential oils to 20 ml carrier oil. *To awaken: add up to 8 drops uplifting essential oils to 20 ml carrier oil.*	To promote sleep: a slow, gentle shoulder massage (see page 58–9) or a relaxing foot and ankle massage (see page 66–7). To revive: a firm, energetic foot massage (see page 66–7) to boost energy.	• *To aid sleep: place 2 drops of calming essential oils on a handkerchief and inhale; or add up to 5 drops of essential oils to the bath.* • *To awaken: place 2 drops of uplifting essential oils on a handkerchief and inhale, or add up to 5 drops of essential oils to the bath.*

ACHES & PAINS

ENERGETIC EXERCISE or repetitive activities such as typing or lifting heavy weights all cause occasional aches and pains. Massage and aromatherapy can reduce pain resulting from tension and overexertion. Both induce relaxation and some essential oils also have analgesic properties. Like exercise, massage is thought to increase the amount of endorphins (pain-relieving hormones) circulating in the body. By stimulating touch and pressure receptors, massage also helps keep information from pain receptors from reaching the brain. The benefits of massage have been recognized since the 10th century, when Avicenna wrote, "As a sequel to athletics, restorative friction produces repose." To make a massage oil blend, choose up to four essential oils from those suggested and blend with a carrier oil to suit your skin type (see page 14).

Choose either German or Roman chamomile (see page 19).

PROBLEM	USEFUL ESSENTIAL OILS		GENERAL EFFECT OF OILS
BACKACHE Including stiffness and pain in the lower back, shoulders, and neck.	Black pepper *Chamomile Eucalyptus Juniper	Lavender Melissa Orange Rosemary	Anti-inflammatory and warming oils help relax aching muscles.
HEADACHE Including tension headaches, migraines, and neuralgia.	*Chamomile Geranium Lavender Marjoram	Peppermint Petitgrain Rose Rosemary	Fresh scents help relieve tension.
LEG CRAMPS Spasmodic gripping pain in the muscles that results from overexertion or exercise.	Clary sage Cypress Juniper Lavender	Marjoram	Penetrating and anti-spasmodic oils relax muscles.
MUSCULAR ACHES & PAINS Resulting from strenuous use of the muscles.	Eucalyptus German chamomile Ginger	Juniper Lavender Marjoram Rosemary	Analgesic and warming oils relax muscles and relieve mild pain and soothe the area.
SPRAINS, STRAINS & SWOLLEN JOINTS Resulting from wrenched, stretched, or over-used muscles, including arthritis and gout.	*Chamomile Cypress Frankincense Juniper	Lavender Marjoram Rosemary	Calming oils with an anti-inflammatory action.
PRE-EXERCISE WARM-UP To relax and prepare the muscles for exercise.	Lemongrass Marjoram Rosemary		Oils keep muscles supple and relax and calm the nerves.
POST-EXERCISE STIFFNESS To relax tight, sore muscles that ache after sports because of a buildup of waste products.	Eucalyptus German chamomile Juniper	Lemongrass Marjoram	Oils combat aching muscles and aid relaxation.

FOR ACHES & PAINS	BEFORE EXERCISE	AFTER EXERCISE
Essential oils	**Essential oils**	**Essential oils**
5 drops lavender	5 drops lavender	3 drops juniper
2 drops each of frankincense and rosemary	2 drops each of rosemary and marjoram	2 drops each of eucalyptus and German chamomile
Carrier oil	**Carrier oil**	**Carrier oil**
20 ml sweet almond	20 ml sweet almond	20 ml sweet almond
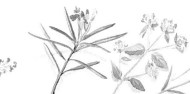	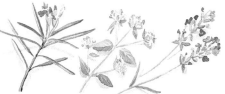	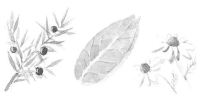

For all three recipes, follow method for basic oil, page 71.

MASSAGE BLEND	**MASSAGE TREATMENT**	**OTHER APPLICATIONS**
Add up to 8 drops essential oils to 20 ml carrier oil.	Firm, soothing massage strokes over the lower back to calm (see pages 48–53). Then gentle circular pressures (see page 46) at the base of the spine, followed by massage around the abdomen.	• *Apply a warm compress (see page 97) made with 2–3 drops of essential oils.* • *Add up to 5 drops of essential oils to the bath.*
Add up to 8 drops essential oils to 20 ml carrier oil.	Shoulder, neck, face, and scalp massage (see pages 56–9) with circular pressures (see page 46) on the temples, forehead, and the base of the skull.	• *Apply a cold compress (see page 97) made with 2 drops of peppermint oil to the forehead.*
Add up to 8 drops essential oils to 20 ml carrier oil.	To release the spasm: rub the leg and pull the foot toward you; hold until the pain passes; then energetically massage the area.	• *Apply a warm compress (see page 97) made with 4 drops of essential oils.* • *If prone to muscle cramps, massaging the blend into the skin regularly can help prevent attacks.*
Add up to 8 drops essential oils to 20 ml carrier oil.	For acute pain: gentle, repetitive massage all over the area to calm it. For persistent pain: firm, rhythmic strokes to stimulate the circulation; and circular pressures (see page 46) on taut muscles.	• *For acute pain: apply a cold compress (see page 97) made with 4 drops of essential oils.* • *For chronic pain: apply a warm compress (see page 97) made with 4 drops of essential oils.*
Add up to 8 drops essential oils to 20 ml carrier oil.	Extremely soft strokes above the site of pain. For example: for a swollen ankle, gentle strokes on the thigh and calf; for a swollen knee, strokes up the thigh toward the lymph nodes of the groin.	• *Apply a cold compress (see page 97) made with 4 drops of essential oils and elevate the limb to prevent swelling.*
Add up to 8 drops essential oils to 20 ml carrier oil.	An energetic full body massage (see pages 48–67) with brisk strokes and kneading (see page 46) on the muscles that will be used most.	• *No other applications advised.*
Add up to 8 drops essential oils to 20 ml carrier oil.	Smooth, rhythmic massage strokes to soothe the whole body, or just on the muscles that have worked hardest, then gentle strokes toward the lymph nodes in the affected area.	• *Add up to 5 drops of essential oils to the bath.*

INFECTIONS & FIRST AID

AMONG OTHER BENEFICIAL QUALITIES, many essential oils have antiseptic, antimicrobial, and anti-inflammatory properties. These oils make useful remedies to treat infections, and respiratory conditions, in particular respond well to them. Eucalyptus and rosemary, for example, have been used traditionally in chest rubs to alleviate the symptoms of influenza and colds. Aromatic oils have been burned as incense to purify the air in sickrooms – with effective results since they kill airborne microbes. I have also found essential oils to be useful first-aid remedies, especially for treating minor burns, cuts, sores, and stings. These remedies are designed for minor ailments and should never replace medical attention. To make a massage oil blend, choose up to four essential oils from those suggested and blend with a carrier oil to suit your skin type (see page 14).

Choose either German or Roman chamomile (see page 19).

PROBLEM	USEFUL ESSENTIAL OILS		GENERAL EFFECT OF OILS
COLDS & COUGHS Including chills, congestion, runny nose, and tickly, inflamed throat.	*Bergamot Cypress Eucalyptus Frankincense Lavender*	*Marjoram Peppermint Rosemary Sandalwood Tea tree*	Oils with antiseptic and antibacterial properties help decongest and ease breathing.
SORE THROAT Including dryness, scratchiness, inflammation, hoarseness, and difficulty swallowing.	*Clary sage Cypress Lavender*	*Peppermint Sandalwood Tea tree*	Soothing and antiseptic oils help fight infection and prevent laryngitis from developing.
MUCUS & NASAL CONGESTION Including inflammation of the mucus membrane, stuffiness, and aching or throbbing around the nose.	*Eucalyptus Frankincense Lavender Peppermint*	*Rosemary Scot's pine Tea tree*	Stimulating, clearing, antiseptic, and soothing oils relieve congestion and discomfort.
CHEST INFECTIONS Including bronchitis and other respiratory problems.	*Cypress Eucalyptus Frankincense Lavender*	*Marjoram Peppermint Sandalwood Tea tree*	Refreshing oils help clear the chest and aid breathing.
EARACHE Aching or pain in the ear.	*Lavender Roman chamomile*	*Tea tree*	Soothing, antiseptic, analgesic, and anti-inflammatory oils ease discomfort.
MINOR CUTS, ABRASIONS & SORES Including scrapes, wounds, abscesses, and boils.	*Bergamot Geranium Lavender*	*Tea tree German chamomile*	Antiseptic oils prevent infection and relieve pain.
MINOR BURNS Including heat burns, scalding, and friction burns.	*Geranium German chamomile*	*Lavender Tea tree*	Soothing and antiseptic oils diminish pain and prevent infection.
INSECT BITES & STINGS Including mosquito, flea, tick, and spider bites, and wasp and bee stings.	**Chamomile Lavender Tea tree*		Soothing oils relieve itching and stinging sensations while reducing swelling.

TO CLEAR THE CHEST

Essential oils
5 drops sandalwood
2 drops each of marjoram
and frankincense
Carrier oil
20 ml sunflower

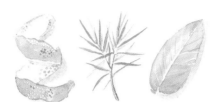

FOR COUGHS & COLDS

Essential oils
4 drops bergamot
2 drops each of tea tree and eucalyptus
Carrier oil
20 ml sunflower

FOR CONGESTION

Essential oils
2 drops each of rosemary and eucalyptus
1 drop Scot's pine
Carrier oil
20 ml sweet almond

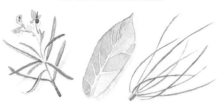

For all three recipes, follow method for basic oil, page 71.

MASSAGE BLEND	MASSAGE TREATMENT	OTHER APPLICATIONS
Add up to 8 drops essential oils to 20 ml carrier oil.	Rhythmic stroking on the chest to soothe the area, followed by a gentle neck and face massage (see pages 56–9) and finally gentle static pressures (see page 46) on either side of the nose.	• *Use 4 drops of essential oils in an inhalation (see page 97).* **Do not use if you have asthma**. • *Add up to 5 drops of essential oils to the bath.* • *Add 5 drops of essential oils to 1 cup of water to make an air freshener (see page 97).*
Add up to 8 drops essential oils to 20 ml carrier oil.	Gentle strokes down the neck; then large, gentle, circular movements on either side of the neck. Finish with softer, more soothing strokes.	• *Apply to the neck a warm compress (see page 97) made with 4 drops of essential oils.*
Add up to 8 drops essential oils to 20 ml carrier oil.	Deep, circular pressures (see page 46) at the base of the skull, followed by squeezing the eyebrows, pressure on the eyebrows, forehead, and base of the nose, and finally gentle strokes down the nose, out to the ears, and down the neck.	• *Use 4 drops of essential oils in an inhalation (see page 97).* **Do not use if you have asthma**. • *Place 2 drops of essential oils on a handkerchief and inhale.*
Add up to 8 drops essential oils to 20 ml carrier oil.	A chest massage (see pages 58–9), including cat stroking (see page 47), gentle stroking, and circular pressures (see page 46). Finish with more gentle stroking.	• *Use 4 drops of essential oils in an inhalation (see page 97).* **Do not use if you have asthma**. • *Add up to 5 drops of essential oils to the bath.*
Add up to 8 drops essential oils to 20 ml carrier oil.	Massage all around the ear and jaw, followed by gentle circular pressures (see page 46) and finally light strokes all over the area.	• ***Do not put essential oils or massage blends in the ear***.
	Massage is inadvisable.	• *Clean affected area with cool, boiled water, then apply a cold compress (see page 97) made with 4 drops of essential oils.*
	Massage is inadvisable.	• *Immerse affected area in cold water then apply neat lavender oil or a cold compress (see page 97) made with 4 drops of lavender oil and 2 of chamomile oil.*
	Massage is inadvisable.	• *Dab a drop of lavender or tea tree on affected area.* • *If swollen, apply a cold compress (see page 97) made with 2 drops each of lavender and chamomile oils.*

DIGESTIVE PROBLEMS

ESSENTIAL OILS AND MASSAGE can help reduce the discomfort and symptoms of digestive problems from which we suffer because of stress, overindulgence, allergy, or food poisoning. Some oils, such as chamomile and lavender, have anti-spasmodic properties and relieve cramps and pain. Peppermint soothes the digestive processes and helps combat flatulence, and mandarin can help restore a lost appetite. Gentle, rhythmic massage of the abdomen reduces tension, relaxes the muscles, and encourages peristalsis, the wavelike movement of food and waste products through the digestive system. If digestive problems persist or become regular, consult a doctor. To make a massage oil blend, choose up to four essential oils from those suggested and blend with a carrier oil to suit your skin type (see page 14).

Choose either German or Roman chamomile (see page 19).

PROBLEM	USEFUL ESSENTIAL OILS		GENERAL EFFECT OF OILS
INDIGESTION Including heartburn, abdominal pain, flatulence, and difficulty in digesting food.	Juniper Lavender Orange Peppermint Roman chamomile	Rosemary	Anti-spasmodic oils soothe the digestive processes.
CONSTIPATION Including bloating, cramps, irregular and difficult bowel movements, and general discomfort.	Black pepper Lemongrass Mandarin Marjoram Orange	Rosemary	Stimulating oils encourage digestion, relax the muscles, and ease tension.
IRRITABLE BOWEL SYNDROME Including abdominal cramps, flatulence, and bloating; may be linked to stress.	*Chamomile Lavender Marjoram Melissa	Neroli Peppermint	Soothing and relaxing oils calm the nerves and reduce stress.
HANGOVER Including nausea, aching body, and headache.	Jasmine Juniper Lavender Peppermint Rose	Rosemary Sandalwood	Refreshing oils ease an aching body and clear the mind.
NAUSEA Including the urge to vomit, motion sickness, and an accompanying loss of appetite.	Ginger Lavender Orange Peppermint Petitgrain		Fresh and relaxing oils help calm the stomach and mind, and relieve nausea and headache.
COLIC & GAS IN BABIES Including pain in the abdomen and flatulence.	Peppermint Roman chamomile		Gentle anti-spasmodic oils soothe the abdomen.

FOR CONSTIPATION	FOR A HANGOVER	FOR INDIGESTION
Essential oils	**Essential oils**	**Essential oils**
4 drops mandarin	5 drops sandalwood	4 drops orange
3 drops citrus oils	3 drops lavender	2 drops Roman chamomile
2 drops rosemary	1 drop jasmine	1 drop peppermint
Carrier oil	**Carrier oil**	**Carrier oil**
20 ml sweet almond	20 ml sweet almond	20 ml sweet almond

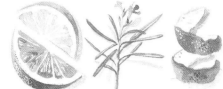 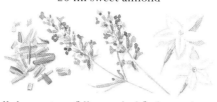 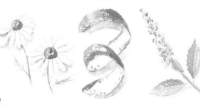

For all three recipes, follow method for basic oil, page 71.

MASSAGE BLEND	MASSAGE TREATMENT	OTHER APPLICATIONS
Add up to 8 drops essential oils to 20 ml carrier oil.	To soothe: slow, gentle clockwise strokes around the abdomen (see pages 62–3). To promote sleep: an abdomen massage followed by a back massage (see pages 48–53), finishing with cat stroking (see page 47) before going to bed.	• *Place 1 drop of peppermint oil on a handkerchief and inhale.*
Add up to 8 drops essential oils to 20 ml carrier oil.	Rhythmic strokes over the abdomen, including undulating pressures (see page 62) in a triangle around the navel, followed by a foot massage (see pages 66–7).	• *Add up to 5 drops of essential oils to the bath.*
Add up to 8 drops essential oils to 20 ml carrier oil.	Gentle massage of the abdomen (see pages 62–3) and, if time permits, a full body massage (see pages 48–67), paying extra attention to areas of tension.	• *Add up to 5 drops of essential oils to the bath.*
Add up to 8 drops essential oils to 20 ml carrier oil.	A gentle face massage, concentrating on the forehead and temples; then a scalp massage using firm, deep circular pressures (see page 46), as if shampooing the hair. Finish with strokes on the base of the skull to relieve tension.	• *Add up to 5 drops of essential oils to the bath.*
	Massage is inadvisable.	• *Place 2 drops of essential oils on a handkerchief and inhale.*
Add up to 2 drops essential oils to 20 ml carrier oil. If the baby is under 3 months, use sweet almond oil alone.	Very gentle strokes over the abdomen in a clockwise direction.	• *No other applications advised.*

WOMEN'S HEALTH

AROMATHERAPY CAN BE OF GREAT BENEFIT throughout a woman's life for both emotional and physical ailments. It gives relief from premenstrual syndrome (PMS) and menstrual cramps, soothes the symptoms of vaginal infections, and eases menopause. Aromatherapy and massage, if used with care, are extremely effective in pregnancy. In pregnancy, always seek advice from a doctor and qualified aromatherapist before using essential oils. During the first three months, do not use essential oils – use sweet almond oil alone for massage. From the fourth month of pregnancy, use very low dilutions of essential oil (1% or less), choosing gentle oils such as those listed on page 16. To make a massage oil blend, choose up to four of your favorite essential oils from those suggested and blend with a carrier oil to suit your skin type (see page 14).

*Choose either German or Roman chamomile (see page 19).

PROBLEM	USEFUL ESSENTIAL OILS		GENERAL EFFECT OF OILS
CYSTITIS Including stinging, burning, and the urge to urinate frequently.	Bergamot Geranium Juniper	Lavender Sandalwood Tea tree	Antiseptic oils help relieve stress and discomfort.
VAGINAL YEAST INFECTIONS May include discharge and/or itching, irritation, and discomfort.	Geranium Juniper Lavender	Sandalwood Tea tree	Antiseptic and antifungal oils help alleviate the condition.
PMS & MENSTRUAL CRAMPS Including bloating, depression, fatigue, irritability, and discomfort.	Clary sage Geranium Jasmine Marjoram	Melissa Roman chamomile Rose	Calming and soothing oils induce relaxation and ease pain, reduce fluid retention, and uplift the mind.
SYMPTOMS OF PREGNANCY Including morning sickness, tension, and backache. **Do not use essential oils in the first 3 months; consult a doctor and qualified aromatherapist.**	*Chamomile Lavender Mandarin Neroli	Peppermint Petitgrain Rose	Refreshing oils soothe and relax.
LABOR Including pain and anxiety.	Clary sage Lavender		Confidence-boosting oils relax and calm, encourage contractions, and ease pain.
POSTPARTUM DEPRESSION Including fatigue and physical exhaustion, lack of energy, and melancholy.	Bergamot Melissa Neroli	Roman chamomile Rose	Uplifting and stress-reducing oils cheer, relax, and pamper.
SYMPTOMS OF MENOPAUSE Including irritability, insomnia, depression, itchy skin, and hot flashes.	Clary sage Frankincense Rose	Roman chamomile Sandalwood	Rich, warm, and feminine-scented oils soothe the skin, balance mood swings, and ease hot flashes.
CELLULITE & STRETCH MARKS Including dimpled, fatty areas on the hips, thighs, or upper arms, and rippled fat resulting from rapid weight gain, such as in adolescence or pregnancy.	CELLULITE Cypress Geranium Juniper Mandarin	STRETCH MARKS Frankincense Geranium Mandarin Neroli	Invigorating oils stimulate the circulation and reduce fluid retention in areas of cellulite; or gentle oils nourish the skin, minimizing stretch marks.

FOR CELLULITE	FOR PMS	FOR STRETCH MARKS
Essential oils	**Essential oils**	**Essential oils**
3 drops each of rosemary, geranium, and juniper	5 drops lavender, 2 drops each of Roman chamomile and geranium	2 drops mandarin
Carrier oil	**Carrier oil**	1 drop each of frankincense and neroli
20 ml sunflower	20 ml sweet almond	**Carrier oils**
		10 ml each of jojoba and avocado

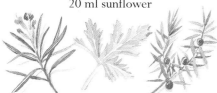 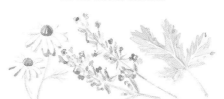 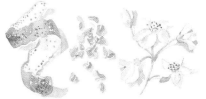

For all three recipes, follow method for basic oil, page 71.

MASSAGE BLEND	MASSAGE TREATMENT	OTHER APPLICATIONS
Add up to 8 drops essential oils to 20 ml carrier oil.	Massage of the lower back and abdomen. Visit a doctor if no improvement within 3 days, or if there is backache, fever, or blood in the urine.	• *Add 4 drops of essential oils to the bath or add 1 drop to a sitz bath and bathe affected area.*
Add up to 8 drops essential oils to 20 ml carrier oil.	Massage of the lower back and abdomen. Visit a doctor if condition does not improve within 3 days.	• *Add 4 drops of essential oils to the bath.* • *Add 2 drops of essential oil to 1 tbsp yogurt with active cultures; apply to affected area.*
Add up to 8 drops essential oils to 20 ml carrier oil.	Soothing massage strokes over the back and abdomen. If time permits, a full body massage (see pages 48–67). Early attention can prevent symptoms from developing.	• *Add 4 to 6 drops of essential oils to a warm bath.* • *Apply a warm compress (see page 97) made with 4 drops of essential oils to the abdomen or breasts.*
First three months: sweet almond oil alone; 4–9 months: 4 drops essential oils to 20 ml carrier oil.	**Do not massage with essential oils in the first 3 months. Do not massage for morning sickness.** To ease discomfort, gently massage around the lower back. Avoid deep pressures.	• *For morning sickness, use 4 drops of essential oils in a vaporizer (see page 97).*
Add up to 8 drops essential oils to 20 ml carrier oil.	Gentle stroking over the lower back and waist, followed by a firm, rhythmic foot massage (see pages 66–7), particularly around the ankle and the ball of the foot, to induce calm.	• *Use 2 drops of essential oil in an inhalation (see page 97). **Do not use if you have asthma.*** • *Add 5 drops of essential oils to 1 cup of water to make an air freshener (see page 97).*
Add up to 8 drops essential oils to 20 ml carrier oil.	A full body massage (see pages 48–67), paying extra attention to the back.	• *Add 5 drops of essential oils to 1 cup of water to make an air freshener (see page 97).* • *Add up to 5 drops of essential oils to the bath.*
Add up to 8 drops essential oils to 20 ml carrier oil.	A relaxing full body massage (see pages 48–67), concentrating on pampering the face.	• *Add up to 5 drops of essential oils to the bath.*
Add up to 8 drops essential oils to 20 ml carrier oil (stretch marks: use 10 ml each of avocado oil and jojoba as carrier oil).	For cellulite: daily brushing (see page 92) and gentle massage, then rhythmic kneading (see page 46) and finally very soft strokes toward the groin. For stretch marks: gentle circular stroking (see page 45).	• *For cellulite: add 4–5 drops of essential oils to the bath.* • *For stretch marks: add 5 drops of essential oils diluted in 10 ml avocado oil or jojoba to the bath.*

SKIN & HAIR PROBLEMS

THE CONDITION OF THE SKIN AND HAIR reflects our basic health. To stay healthy, skin requires a nourishing diet, including lots of fresh fruit and vegetables and plenty of water, as well as regular exercise and enough sleep. The skin is closely connected with the nervous system and is sensitive to changes in our emotions. Stress increases the likelihood of acne, cold sores, and other skin problems, and massaging with nourishing scented oils is of great benefit. It is important to treat even minor skin complaints carefully and gently, and essential oils are ideal, with their healing, antiseptic, and anti-inflammatory properties. Hair also benefits from pampering with massage and conditioning oils. To make a massage oil blend, choose up to four essential oils from those suggested and blend with a carrier oil to suit your skin type (see page 14).

Choose either German or Roman chamomile (see page 19).

PROBLEM	USEFUL ESSENTIAL OILS		GENERAL EFFECT OF OILS
ACNE Irritated, inflamed pimply skin, including the stress that accompanies the condition.	Bergamot *Chamomile Geranium Juniper	Lavender Lemongrass Petitgrain Tea tree	Antiseptic oils help reduce inflammation.
BROKEN CAPILLARIES Dilated or broken thread veins on the skin, especially noticeable on the face.	*Chamomile Cypress Frankincense	Geranium Rose	Oils calm and strengthen the skin while encouraging the veins to constrict.
COLD SORES Blisters on or near the mouth that may burn and tingle.	Bergamot *Chamomile Melissa	Tea tree	Antiviral oils reduce swelling and promote healing.
ECZEMA & PSORIASIS Red, scaly patches on the skin, accompanied by itching and discomfort.	Cypress Frankincense Geranium Juniper	Lavender Sandalwood German chamomile	Calming and anti-inflammatory oils ease itching and soreness and promote healing.
VARICOSE VEINS Dilated veins that may protrude from the skin and be accompanied by pain and discomfort.	Cypress Geranium Orange		Soothing and astringent oils ease inflammation.
DRY HAIR Including brittle, lifeless hair with split ends.	*Chamomile Jasmine Rosemary Sandalwood		Gentle oils improve texture and increase shine.
DANDRUFF Including dry, itchy scalp and flaking skin.	Cypress Juniper Lavender Mandarin	Rosemary	Cleansing and antiseptic oils help improve the condition of the scalp.
HEAD LICE Including intense itching resulting from infestation.	Geranium Lavender Lemon	Rosemary Tea tree	Antiseptic oils ease scalp irritation and rid it of lice.

SKIN TONIC

Essential oils
10 drops each of German chamomile
and petitgrain, 4 drops tea tree
Base
10 ml vodka, 100 ml distilled water

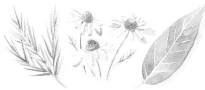

*Follow method for basic aromatic vinegar,
page 72.*

HAIR CONDITIONER

Essential oils
3 drops sandalwood
2 drops geranium, 1 drop jasmine
Carrier oils
10 ml each of avocado and jojoba

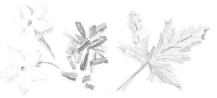

Follow method for basic oil, page 71.

VINEGAR HAIR RINSE

Essential oils
2 drops each of rosemary and lavender
1 drop juniper
Base
5 ml cider vinegar, 10 ml distilled water

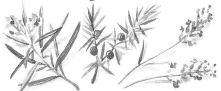

*Follow method for basic aromatic vinegar,
page 72.*

MASSAGE BLEND	**MASSAGE TREATMENT**	**OTHER APPLICATIONS**
Add up to 8 drops essential oils to 20 ml carrier oil.	**If very inflamed, do not massage**. A face massage (see pages 56–7) to increase circulation and lymphatic flow, followed by a toner (see page 72) and a face mask (see page 73).	• *If very inflamed, apply a cold compress (see page 97) made with 4 drops of essential oils.* • *Clean and cool the skin with skin tonic (see above).* • *Dab a drop of tea tree on a cotton swab on pimples.*
Add 1–2 drops essential oils to 10 ml wheat-germ or sweet almond oil.	Gentle massage over the skin, using smooth, soft movements. Avoid energetic strokes.	• *Apply a cold compress (see page 97) made with 4 drops of essential oils.*
	Massage is inadvisable.	• *Dilute essential oil to 1% in carrier oil (see page 15) and dab on the cold sore with a cotton swab.*
Do a patch test (see page 16) and if no reaction, add up to 8 drops essential oils to 20 ml carrier oil.	Plenty of gentle, rhythmic strokes over the back (see pages 48–53) to improve morale and relieve stress.	• *Do a patch test (see page 16) to ensure essential oils will not cause an adverse reaction, then add up to 5 drops of essential oils to the bath.*
Add up to 8 drops essential oils to 20 ml carrier oil.	Gently massage around the varicose vein, **but never on the vein itself**. To prevent varicose veins, massage the legs and feet (see pages 54–5 and 64–7) two or three times a week.	• *Apply a cold compress (see page 97) made with 4 drops of essential oils, and elevate the legs.* • *Add 4 drops of essential oils to a cold footbath.*
Add 6 drops essential oils to 10 ml each of avocado oil and jojoba, then heat over a pan of hot water.	Massage warm blend into the hair and scalp with firm, circular movements. Stroke to the ends of the hair. Leave for 15 minutes, then wash with unscented shampoo.	• *Apply vinegar hair rinse (see above) after shampooing.* • *Once a week, apply hair conditioner (see above), leave for 3–10 minutes and then shampoo.*
Add 3 drops essential oils to 10 ml jojoba.	Massage the oil into the whole scalp, with large circular pressures (see page 46) to loosen dead scaly skin and prevent further buildup of dandruff.	• *Add 5 drops of essential oils to 10 ml unscented shampoo and wash as normal; repeat for several weeks.* • *After shampooing, use a final rinse of 5 ml vinegar, 10 ml water, and 3 drops of rosemary oil.*
	Massage is inadvisable.	• *Add 10 drops of essential oils to 10 ml jojoba. Work through hair with a fine-toothed comb. If scalp is irritated, rub in and leave overnight; rinse the next day.*

INDEX

USEFUL ADDRESSES

Local health food stores are generally good places to look for supplies plus free brochures and publications listing services, organizations, and other sources pertaining to aromatherapy massage.

Stores & Suppliers

Aphrodisia
264 Bleeker Street
New York, New York 10014
(212) 989-6440
Mail orders accepted

Atlantis Rising
7909 SE Stark
Portland, Oregon 97215
(503) 254-7555
Mail orders accepted

Aveda
Aveda Customer Relations
(800) 328-0849
Call for location of store
nearest you

The Body Shop
(800) 984-0035
Call for location of store
nearest you

Organic Market
229 Seventh Avenue
New York, New York 10011
(212) 645-8730

Mail order suppliers

Caswell Massey Company Ltd.
100 Enterprise Place
Dover, Delaware 19901
(800) 326-0500

Herb Products Company
P.O. Box 898
North Hollywood, California
91601
(818) 984-3141

Les Herbes
9 Gerry Lane
Huntington, New York 11743
(516) 271-4246

Lotus Light
P.O. Box 1008
Silver Lake, Wisconsin 53170
(800) 548-3824

The Body Shop by Mail
45 Horsehill Road
Cedar Knolls, New Jersey 07927
(800) 984-0035

Information & research

American Botanical Council
P.O. Box 201660
Austin, Texas 78720
(512) 331-8868

American Massage Therapy
Association (AMTA)
820 Davis Street Suite 100
Evanston, Illinois 60201-4444
(312) 761-2682

Herb Research Foundation
1007 Pearl Street, Suite 200
Boulder, Colorado 80302
(303) 449-2265

Education & training

The American Institute for
Aromatherapy & Herbal Studies
9 Gerry Lane
Huntington, New York 11743
(516) 271-4246

California School of
Herbal Studies
P.O. Box 39
Forrestville, California 95436
(707) 887-7457

New York Open Center, Inc.
A Nonprofit Holistic Learning
Center
83 Spring Street
New York, New York 10012
(212) 219-2527

The New Center for Wholistic
Health Education & Research
6801 Jericho Turnpike
Syosset, New York 11791-4413
(800) 922-7337
(516) 364-0808

ACKNOWLEDGMENTS

AUTHOR'S ACKNOWLEDGMENTS
I would like to thank everyone who helped, and especially Rhiannon Lewis of The Aromatherapy Database for the latest research on essential oils and for checking the text; Hilda Butler CChem FRSC BSc (SpChem) BSc (ApBiol), for all her help and advice; Dr. Cao Bei, of the Section of Rehabilitation, Beijing University of Traditional Chinese Medicine, Beijing, for information on the use of essential oils in China; Hakim Naimuddin Zubairy, Director of Research Bait al Hikmat (The House of Wisdom), Hamdard University, Karachi, for information on essential oils in India and Pakistan; Der Pao Graham, Dame Gilberte Brunsdon-Lenaerts, and Begum Kishwa Rizwi for their many kindnesses; Dr. Peter Wilde BSc, PhD, FRSC, for information on rose oil and details of the Phytonic process; to all my colleagues, clients, and students for all their suggestions and encouragement, especially Carola

Beresford-Cooke, Jackie Pietroni, Amina Shah and Anne Vadgama for checking text; Gill Whitworth for her encouragement and enthusiasm and for holding the fort while I was submerged in paper; everyone at Dorling Kindersley, especially Helen Townsend and Jo Grey; and finally Sandra Lousada for her beautiful photographs.

PUBLISHERS ACKNOWLEDGMENTS
Dorling Kindersley would like to thank the following: Beverley Vas at Splitz, Theatrical Hosiery Company, London, SW4, for the clothing; Elizabeth David Cookshop; French, Flint & Ormco Ltd.; Reads Nursery; Royal Botanic Gardens, Kew; Royal Botanical Gardens, Sydney; Royal Horticultural Society, Wisley.
Models: Charlie P. at Models 1 Men, Dorte Jensen, Helen Gatward, Sharon Caines, Karen Su Ying Woo, Hanna Andrews at Models 1, Lucy Berridge.

Make-up: Barbara Jones, Ya'nina and Ellen Kramer from Artistic Licence.
Editorial assistance: Lorna Damms, Roddy Craig, Charlotte Evans, Camela Decaire.
Index: Michèlle Clarke.

PICTURE CREDITS :
Key to pictures:
t = top; c = center; b = bottom; l = left; r = right
Photography by Sandra Lousada except:
Tim Ridley 1, 4, 7, 8-9, 10, 14-5, 16c, 17tr, 18tr, 19tr, 20c, 20cr, 21,22tr, 23tr, 24tr, 25tr, 26tr, 27tr, 28tr, 29tr, 30tr, 31, 32tr, 33tr, 34tr, 35tr, 36, 37tr, 70-1, 72-3; Steve Gorton 27c, 30c, 34c, 35c; Kim Saunders 22c,29c, Peter Anderson 23c; Mary Evans Picture Library 11; Fragonard Parfumeur 13r; Pictures Colour Library Ltd. 12-13.
Illustrations: Charlotte Weiss 4-color plant illustrations; Karen Cochrane arrow artworks and essential oil note artworks.